A Psychiatrists Insights

Henry Veit MD
Distinguished Life
Fellow APA

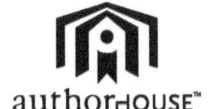

authorHOUSE™

1663 Liberty Drive, Suite 200
Bloomington, Indiana 47403
(800) 839-8640
www.AuthorHouse.com

First published by AuthorHouse 12/22/05

ISBN: 1-4259-1164-1 (e)
ISBN: 1-4208-8165-5 (sc)

Library of Congress Control Number: 2005908196

Printed in the United States of America
Bloomington, Indiana

This book is printed on acid-free paper.

Chapter 1
My Life as a medical Doctor

In recalling my childhood, I go back to 2 ½ years of age. That was when I was smuggled across the Russia border in a feather tick mattress into Poland- My father, who had been a staff officer in General Kerensky's Army was fighting Communism. My Grandfather had already been executed by the Communists and all his worldly possessions amounting to about 100 million in American dollars was confiscated. Fortunately gold coins, buried in the flower bed of the old homestead were dug up by my father, to bribe the Russian Border Guards so that my mother, aunt, my father, and myself would cross into Poland. We traveled to Homburg, Germany. My uncle Heinrich in millwaukee, Wis sent money to my father, so in 1922 we came to America going directly to Milwaukee, Wis. We were Volga Germans- people who migrated from Austria and Germany into Russia during the time of Catherine the great. Hence farms and small communities developed along the Volga river in the Saratof, Russia area.

My father of Austrian descent, survived World War I but as an officer he was captured and kept in Finland for almost a year, before the war ended. Then he returned home only to end up in the war against communism. He spoke Russian, German, Polish, and Finnish. And upon coming to the U.S.A. he also picked up English. My mother was born in Poland of German parents who were gentlemen farmers but with World War II got pushed into the war.

Dad was enthusiatic about coming to the U.S.A. democracy. He had no problem in finding work in a bakery. My mother went to work for North Western Life Ins. as a cleaning woman.

When I first went to the public school, age 5, I had problems with speaking English. German was the home language. My first teacher thought that I was stupid, but in due time I mastered the English Language. I was so interested in learning, that I went to summer school to get advanced grading. By the age of 16, I graduated from High School- I did spend the 4th thorough the 6th grade at a Lutheran Parochial School and that may have contributed me to strong studying, my grades ranged betweens A's and B's. In Junior High School as I was helpful to "slower learning classroom friends, I was nicknamed Professor, and being near-sighted with thick lenses, these friends were protective of me on the playground.

Teachers and Librarians, and others in my life took an interest in me, and really stimulated me, so I progressed readily in my studies. The local librarian recommended books for me to read, Shakespeare's works, war and peace, when I was only 12 years old. The English teacher had me join her Shakespeare club. All these helped me intellectually. As I grew up in a "rough neighborhood" I had to learn to defend myself. At the age of 14, the Milwaukee Champion Amateur Boxer, who lived nearby took an interest in me. In time no one even tried to get rough with me. Also the Science High School teacher had me stay after school twice weekly to do genetic studies on fruit flies.

A Lutheran Pastor, to whose church our family went every Sunday, played strong role in my future. In one of his family visits, he disparaged our family as being serfs. This Pastor also believed and stated that God "spoke through him", The factors made my Dad change churches and transferred me from Lutheran church school, to the Public Junior High School.

By the year 1928, my dad was able to buy a small home near where we rented. It became easier to visit with neighbors, as my grass cutting and shoveling snow for them was considered neighborly. I was interested in joining the Boy Scouts, but the rigid Missouri Synod prohibited that. By the way Dancing, Card playing, and movies were also not acceptable. As time went on, church affiliation changed, so less strict rules were manifested.

In the Thirties. no scholarships were available. Hence, to pay college tuition, I worked as a janitor, then as a bartender, and finally in Medical School as First Aid and office manager. There was no time left for fooling around, no dating, just work and studying until age 21. I was starting my Junior year in Medical school with more clinical work and less book work then. Graduating at age 23, I was the youngest in the class.

Little did I realize an internship in 1943 would be exhausting. The 24 hour shifts on and 12 hours off. finally wears one down. But, finally one in love gets one over the exhaustion. So July 17, 1943. I got married to a wonderful, lovely nurse, and our marriage lasted almost 58 years before she died. Our honeymoon was a weekend at Wisconsin Dells, Wis. But, as an intern, my room and board place was at the Hospital. I shall never forget my O.B/Gyn. Internship – delivering babied at the hospital and at the Salvation Army for unmarried mother. It is hard to believe that I attended over 200 births, with fortunately not a single casualty. Most of these births seems to occur at night, so I decided that specialty was not for me.

During 1936, with repeal of Prohibition my parents were able to purchase a small restaurant-bar combination on the first floor, and living quarters on the second floor. My folks were able to quit their jobs, and concentrate on running the business successfully. There I did the early morning janitor work from age 17-21, and then I tried bartending. The last was a great experience, as it made me decide not to smoke, drink, or consider dating any strange female –especially those at the bar! Love at first sight first occurred at age 23, as an intern at St. Josephs Hospital in Milwaukee, Wis. The second shift nurse came out and relieved the nurse assisting me, and there she was. I was age 24 and she was 25, when we married.

I went into Military Service -1st, Lt. Medical Corp, Jan. 13, 1944, my wife was able to accompany me to all my appointments- Atlantic City Military Hospital for returning injured army personnel, then New York City to Columbia University.- Neurology and psychiatric Institute, where I became an Army Military Neuro-psychiatrist. Our first child- Kirk was born on Governors Is. at an Army Hospital. From there, I was transferred to Camp Claiborne, La. Where I managed a psychiatric ward – and later the psychiatric Dept. of three wards. From there, I was transferred to Fort Smith, Ark. where I was the Medical Administrator of an 800 bed Army Hospital. This last job I held from Jan. 46-Aug.46, when I was discharged with the ending of War World II. I was never able to be promoted to the rank of Colonel as the war was ending during my time, as the two officers before me were colonels.

Interestingly, I was accepted to return to Columbia University – Neurology and Psychiatric Institute to finish my specialty training for civilian Neuro-psychiatry. An offer was also made by a visiting Neuropsychiatrist, Dept. Chief of Neuropsychiatry at Colorado School of Medicine, Denver Colorado. The latter had published a college textbook on psychiatry by Strecker and Ebough. The latter person influenced me to go to Denver. After the first year realizing he had the need to have his residents write his talks and also add his name to their articles – I couldn't "stomach" staying any longer. So my final year was completed by me at Milwaukee County General Hospital. affiliated with the teaching colleagues at Marquette School of Medicine. After completing my requirements in Neuropsychiatry Specialty, I progressed to ending up on the Marquette School of Medicine Faculty for 14 years.

With part-time Teaching of two subjects- Neurology and Psychiatry, I developed private practice in order to have an income. In the late 40, 50's and early 60's, no part-time faculty member was paid, as it was, at that time considered an Honor to be appointed. However, my teaching at the Medical School was ended by me, when the Dean asked me, and four other faculty members to tutor the lower grade students admitted as the result of Federal Money donated to such administrators. All five of us resigned! Hence, The Dean had to work out other arrangements. This occurred in all the other Medical Colleges in the U.S.A. My view, and shared by the other four if we tutor these people so they can graduate, who will tutor them to keep up with the advancements in medicine later on..

Fortunately, with leaving being a Consulting Psychiatrist for the State of Wis., Milwaukee County General Hospital, and a private local Sanitarium, my time was well used. In due time I was able to establish a clinic (Medical Service Corporation) with two other psychiatrists, two psychologists, and two social workers. For spiritual guidance at the clinic, a rabbi, catholic priest, and a pastor volunteered some time. This proved to be most therapeutic. In due time, corporations in Milwaukee, North Western Mutual life, Miller Corp., Briggs and Stratton requested consultations for these employees. Getting to know and helping individual persons was enjoyable and rewarding. In fact, when I closed the clinic (as both of my associates had died, and finding satisfactory replacements was difficult) I was treating their generation descendents. That was my first retirement.

Moving up to the northern part of Wis. to our summer place, I was persuaded to go into a private Neuropsychiatric practice again, by two former students of mine, who were General practitioners in the area. Over the years, I had picked up a Michigan, Minn., California, Arizona, licenses in addition, so I was able to practice in Michigan's Northern Peninsula. After developing two

County Counseling centers, and a psychiatric wing in Menominee Mich. Hosp, other psychiatrists arrived, so that I could retire there after seven years. Over the years, I had 32 medical articles on Neurology and psychiatry published in Medical Journals in the U.S.A., Europe, and South America.

As the good lord gave me 58 years as a licensed M.D. in Wis., I feel driven to write this book for the benefit of the lay public, hence I will avoid as much as I can the Medical technology. As psychiatry has only recently been accepted by the Medical Profession and the public as an emotional illness factor, I hope to enlighten the understanding of more people.

So, first – What can be considered an emotional stable person. So I will present my view first, then that of a much – honored doctor – William c. Menninger M.D.

Chapter 2
What is well adjusted person in the U.S.A.?

In the U.S.A., this person represents the threefold ideal of duty honor, and Country a principle by which to live and serve! To achieve this, are needed the moral principles that sustain the philosophy of America, and freedom as set forth in the opening paragraph of the Declaration of Independence. That philosophy regards men as a creature of God. As such, each person is accountable and responsible to his career for the way he or she performs their duty duties, maintain their honor, and serve their family, community and country.

Duty concerns personal responsibility for your assigned task at work, at home, and in your community. You will do the best of your ability, do the task assigned, as part of the team, for your own and everyone's welfare.

That is a measure of your conscience – knowing what is right and what is wrong. Unfortunately, in our imperfect world, there are persons born without the ability to develop a conscience. Duty may require routine hardships, and even sacrifice.

Honor signifies the sense of what is right, just and true along with a way of life as related to social needs

Honor, as a prescription of bottle of medicine would be:

RX: promises kept – 1 oz

Duty done – 1 oz

Courage – sufficient mix to see things through

The ideal of Country requires emphasis on the moral greatness of the history and traditions of our country, for then only can service and sacrifice in defense of our way of life can be worthwhile. Hence, we must have an accepted common culture, one common neutral out look on life, and one common language (English). We need the common traditions to keep us fused into one single coomunity.

In his approach, William C. Menninger M.D. (1899-1966) presented seven criteria for an emotionally stable, well-adjusted person! These are:

1 the ability to deal constructively with reality.

2 The capacity to adapt to change.

3 A relative freedom from symptoms that are produced by tension and anxieties.

4 The capacity to find more satisfaction in giving than receiving.

5 The capacity to relate to other people in a consistent manner with mutual satisfaction and helpfulness.

6 The capacity to sublimate, and to direct ones instinctive hostile energy into creative and constructive outlets

7. The capacity to love and accept being loved.

Chapter 3
OUTLINE FOR MENTAL STATUS EXAMINATIONS

I. ATTITUDE AND GENERAL BEHAVIOR

Note: It is best to write or dictate this division at the conclusion of the examination, inasmuch as it should include a description of what is observed *during the interview*.

A. Preliminary Description

Brief description of what nurses, attendants, physicians and others in contact with the patient have observed, including a brief note of the physical condition.

B. General Description

1. Dress – neat, untidy, appropriate, eccentric, etc.

2. Posture – erect, rigid, changing, tense, relaxed, recumbent, voluntary, constrained, passive, etc.

3. Facial expression – fixed, mobile, masked, ecstatic, suspicious, manneristic, dissociated, stc.

4. Attitude – friendly, genial, cooperative, resistive, negativistic, etc.

5. General mood – calm, elated, depressed, anxious, perplexed, fearful, etc.

6. Motor activity – under or over activity, restlessness, stereotypy, occupational preoccupation, retardation, etc.

MENTAL STATUS

II. STREAM OF TALK AND MENTAL ACTIVITY

A. Talk (Obtained verbatim samples of speech).

1. Form and Quantity – conversational, logical, distractable, flighty, irrelevant, rambling, incoherent, hesitant, interrupted, scattered, blocking, word-salad, verbigeration, neologistic, repetitive, confabulatory, echolalic, over or under-talkative, verbose, circumstantial, garrulous, mute, etc.

2. Rate – under pressure, increased pressure, accelerated, retarded, blocked, etc.

3. Quality – rhyming, punning, alliterative, dramatic, protestive, declamatory, sarcastic, bitter, humorous, witty, ironical, whispering, mumbling, loud, shouting, screaming, singing, whistling, telegrammatic, etc.

B. Psychomotor Activity. (In greater detail than in the first division).

1. Increased activity – maniacal flight, restlessness, stereotypy, bizarre movements, automatisms, fumbling, etc.

2. Reduced activity (note dressing, walking, and performance of tasks) – loss of initiative, lack of spontaneity, bradyphrenia. Is inhibition content-determined (topical) or diffuse? To test have patient count as quickly as possible at various times of day and in varying situations.

MENTAL STATUS

III. EMOTIONAL REACTION

Note: One should gather objective and subjective data and use the question-answer method for the latter. Note the compatibility of mood to the content of thought and the expression of motor activity. Conclude with summary of pertinent findings.

A. Objective

Is the patient composed, complacent?

Irritable, angry?

Happy, elated, exalted?

Boastful, self-satisfied, expansive?

Suspicious, distant, aloof?

Depressed, sad, hopeless?

Anxious, tense, fearful, perplexed?

Indifferent, apathetic, dissociated?

Labile, or markedly unstable?

Is mood appropriate to ideas?

Are there somatic evidences of flushing, tachycardia, perspiration, tears?

What is the accompanying facial expression?

Is depression content-determined (topical) or diffuse?

B. Subjective

How are you?

How do you feel?

How are your spirits?

Do you find it difficult to start new things?

Is it necessary to increase your effort to accomplish your usual tasks?

What do you mean by blue?

Are you frightened?

Do you feel as if you are in a panic?
Do you become angry or irritable?
When? Where? Why?
Have you any ups and downs?
What part of the day is most pleasant?
Least pleasant?
Have you any aches or pains?
How is your appetite, digestion, sleep, weight?
Is life worth living?
Do you feel despondent?
Led to despair?
Rather end life than continue feeling as you do?
Overt suicidal attempts?

MENTAL STATUS

IV. MENTAL TREND: CONTENT OF THOUGHT

Note: Patient should be allowed to tell his story spontaneously. However, it is usually necessary to supplement this by the question and answer method of interrogation and examination.

A. Obsessions, Compulsions

Are you aware of thoughts that you are unable to control or rid yourself of?

Do you fear storms, heights, crowds, traffic?

Is it difficult to come to a decision?

Are you compelled to follow rituals in dressing, walking, speaking, etc.

Do you feel tense if the above are not done?

What do they mean?

B. Feelings of Unreality and Depersonalization

Illusion of false recognition (Déjà vu)

Do persons and objects appear strange to you?

Do you feel as if you were in a fog?

Are you aware of a change in yourself?

Do you feel your identity lost?

Do you feel unnatural?

Is time or space distorted?

C. Delusions. (Gradual approach)

Have you had any unusual, unpleasant, or perplexing experiences?

Have you had any peculiar thoughts, imaginations, or dreams?

D. Persecutory Trends (From ideas of reference to persecutory paranoid delusions).

Are you considered friendly or popular?

Do you enjoy the company of others?

Do people treat you well?

Do they refer to you by changes in facial expression, side glances, or mumblings?

Do they talk about you?

Do they hold grudges against you?

Are you suspicious of others?

Are you inclined to see meanings in all things?

Are you jealous of mate, parents, children, friends?

Do you feel wronged, annoyed, robbed, poisoned?

How do you explain it?

E. Passivity Feelings (From ideas of influence to frank delusional formation)

Do you feel your thoughts or actions controlled by others?

Do people read your mind?

Are your thoughts taken away from you?

Is your mind or body influenced by machines, electricity, mind-reading, hypnotism, or telepathy?

How do you explain it?

F. Somatic Trends (From hypochondriacal ideas to somatic delusions)

What is your health, strength?

Have you any aches or pains?

How is your appetite, digestion, excretory function?

Are you conscious of your heart beat?

What is your sexual power?

What is the condition of your blood?

What does it mean?

G. Self-condemnatory Trends (From increased self-criticism to frank self-condemnatory delusions)

Are you apt to be self-critical?

Do you feel inferior to others?

Do you condemn yourself for the mistakes of others?

Do you feel you have made irreparable errors?

Do you feel your soul is lost?

What does it mean?

Do you feel as if you have committed an unpardonable sin?

What is your financial status?

H. Expansive Trends (From increased self-confidence to frank expansive delusions)

Are you confident of yourself?

Do you feel superior to others?

Have you any unusual powers?

Have you great physical strength, brilliant mind, tremendous wealth?

Are you of high birth?

Have you a special mission in life?

Have you great sexual attraction?

I. Illusions

Have you misinterpreted shadows or noises?

Do body sensations lead you to think you are being touched?

J. Hallucinations

1. Auditory

Do you hear buzzing in your ears?

Noises? Voices?

Where? When? On what occasions?

Are they subdued, loud, clear?

Men's or women's voices?

Do you recognize them?

What do they say?

Are they unpleasant, pleasant?

How do you explain it?

2. Visual

Do you imagine you see things as if in a dream?

Are your eyes open or shut?

At night or in the day?

Where? On what occasions?

What is the attitude of the things you see to you?

What does it mean?

3. Gustatory

Does everything taste normal?

Have you any peculiar tastes?

Sour? Bitter? Metallic?

Does your food taste as if it were tempered?

4. Olfactory

Are you bothered by queer odors?

Are you forced to bathe frequently?

Have you smelled ether or gas?

5. Organic

Do you feel any pressures, tingling, or numbness?

Bones broken? Brain dried up?

Any queer sexual sensations?

Feelings of electricity, vibration?

6. Motor

Do you feel any change in your body position?

Do you have queer sensations from muscles or joints?

MENTAL STATUS

V. SENSORIUM, MENTAL GRASP, AND CAPACITY

Note: Use question and answer method. Avoid abrupt questioning inasmuch as patient usually feels annoyed at having his "mind" tested.

A. Orientation

Date? Day of week, month and time of day?

What place is this?

What is it for?

Where is it located?

What city?

Examiner's name?

Does patient identify nurses, attendants, patients?

B. Memory

1. Remote

Where were you born?

Date of birth?

Age at present?

Year began school?

Year left school?

Year married?

When began work.

Birth date of children?

2. Recent

Where do you live? Address? City? State?

How long have you lived there?

When to hospital? With whom?

How did you come to hospital?

What did you have for dinner yesterday?

How many meals have you had today?

C. Retention and Recall. (Avoid patterns of digits: give 1 digit per second).

Have patient repeat three to ten digits forward after the examiner.

Have him repeat three to eight digits in reverse as given by examiner.

Have patient recall address, color, flower, immediately, 5 min., 1 hour, and 1 day if possible.

D. Counting and Calculation. (Note time required for answer and describe effort made by patient).

Ask the patient to count 1 to 20 as rapidly as possible.

To count backward from 20 to 1.

To do simple multiplication, addition, subtraction, division.

To do simple interest problems.

To subtract successive 7's from 100. (This is also a test for active attention).

E. Grasp of General Information

Ask questions in respect to general historical, geographical, political, and economic import.

Current events and personalities.

F. Reading, Writing, and Speech

The "Cowboy" or other stories should be read by the patient and the examiner should note the character of the reading (facile, laboured, words mispronounced or omitted) and should record the patient exactly.

Does the patient understand story and retain details?

Are there confabulatory trends of irrelevant details?

Have patient write name, address and sentence.

Is the writing free, show, constrained?

Does it show tremor, elisions or transpositions of letters or syllables?

Give patient test phrases to repeat and note character of speech defect, if present.

G. Intelligence

1. Clinical estimate

2. Tests (to be used if there is evidence that patient is subnormal).

a. Children – Stanford Revision of Binet-Simon Test. Kuhlman Test. Performance Tests. (Pintner-Patterson).

b. Adults – Stanford Revision of Binet-Simon Test. Army Alpha Test. Otis Group Test.

H. Judgment. (This is the most difficult division of the examination to test thoroughly. The most valuable means is to gain insight of the patient in his actual situation).

1. Discriminations

Absurdity tests, ball and field tests.

The Binet-Simon Differences (Lie, mistake, etc.)

Abstractions, theoretical situations

2. Actual Situation

Good or poor judgment in general activity.

Judgment better on impersonal than on personal matters.

Plans for the future.

I. Insight

1. Subjective (verbatim statement of patients formulation of himself in his present situation).

Is anything wrong with you?

Has there been a change in you?

Is there anything wrong with your memory or thinking?

Do you feel your difficulty is within you?

Do you feel you need treatment?

What explanation have you for your trouble?

2. Objective

a. Statement of insight as to the emotional nature of illness.

b. Insight into etiological and pathologenetic factors.

Chapter 4
THE MENTAL MECHANISMS

There are a large number of devices by which the personality automatically protects or defends itself against threats. In general, these are reactions to crises or disturbances in inter-personal relationships. People are pushed into defensive reactions by their own unacceptable impulses, particularly sexual and hostile or destructive feelings, ideas, and urges. They arise in situations where the person's wishes and drives are incapable of fulfillment because of frustrations imposed by the person himself or by someone else on whom the person is dependent for love, approval, and security. These wishes and desires usually consist of retained infantile, pleasure-seeking needs, inappropriate to the chronological age of the person.

The aim of the defensive reactions (mental mechanisms) is to reduce anxiety tension (i.e. to diminish distress), to re-establish a façade of self-esteem, and to achieve a measure of gratification despite the imposed frustrations. The following is a list of the most common of these reactions:

1. Wit, humor clowning – The psychological formula is: "I am not distressed in this situation; I am not afraid of it; I can laugh at it." This type of behavior is used as a protection by individuals who feel extremely awkward in a situation, who find it difficult to be with other people, who are afraid of being rejected. Witty behavior may cover up their distress. They may use cynicism and wit to guard against intrusion into their private worlds which are full of trouble and worry. Clowning may be resorted to by boys who are much distressed by their feelings of being ridiculed, rejected, and humiliated because of stoutness or deformity, for example. The clowning covers up distress, but it accomplishes more: They retain contact with and obtain the affection of their friends.

2. Blaming others – The formula is: "I am not to be blamed for failure. Others around me are." The patient makes a mistake in his work because of serious emotional problems, but blames the condition under which he has to work; a man is impotent and blames the women.

3. Attempted justification – (Rationalization, self-vindication) – The psychological motif in rationalization is: "I am not afraid; I am not guilty; I have no conflict because what I have done has a sensible, rational purpose." Two kinds of devices are involved here; the second is more serious than the first. The first merely attempts to make the patient's behavior appear rational so that he can escape humiliation and ridicule and self-contempt. Thus a patient may have complicated conflicts and fears about asserting himself, about having initiative, about getting close to people. He will not recognize and admit this fact, but will instead give such reasons as "It doesn't pay to strive too hard. One is safest alone. In this way I can't be taken advantage of," etc. The second type of device is seen when a patient rationalizes engaging in an activity which disturbs someone else. For example, a superior who hounds his subordinates may give the need for efficiency as the reason for his behavior; the mother who dominates and tortures her child may give her interest and love for him as the reason for her behavior.

4. *Substitution and displacement* – Substitution and displacement are very similar. Substitution usually refers to using another bodily organ instead of the one which affords feared or condemned (Usually genital) gratification. Displacement more frequently refers to emotional reactions or general activities in which the individual responds emotionally to a situation which is in reality different from the one to which he is genuinely reacting.

A severe form of substitution was shown by a married woman, who instead of retiring with her husband, derived genuine erotic pleasure from picking and grooming the skin of her back and face for hours at a time.

Any part of the body or any article of clothing may be substituted for the genital organs in this type of substitute activity. Instances of fetishism belong here, as when a person gets all his pleasure from being aroused and gratified by shoes which belong to the person he desires.

Most complicated forms of substitution are seen in the following: The individual is afraid of genuine emotional attachment, or self-assertion, or final commitment to what he wants to undertake. Whenever situations arise in which he would like to do a certain thing or in which he is requested to do it, he withdraws and masturbates or engages in elaborate fantasies of self-aggrandizement. His formula is: "This way I am safe and I get some enjoyment out of life." it is obvious that such measures are highly complex and involve the individual's image of himself, of other people, and of his activity. This device serves the further purpose of solace as well as substitute activity.

5. *Revival of earlier forms of behavior (regression)* – A good illustration of this type of phenomenon is the recurrence of enuresis (bed-wetting) in children. A child who is well trained in cleanliness may start wetting his bed again when a difficult situation arises. Such a situation is frequently the birth of another child. The older child, who previously felt secure, now feels seriously threatened in regard to the affection and love of his parents. The bed-wetting is partly a direct expression of anxiety, partly an attempt to show his need of parental attention and help, and partly an attempt to be a helpless infant and thus get all of the parent's affection. In such a situation a child may also want the bottle or the breast again.

The revival of earlier goals or of earlier modes of solution is at time equally obvious in the adult. It is manifest in some aspects of his outlook on life, in his fantasies and dreams, as one part of his reaction to situations of stress. Instead of enuresis, the adult may have bladder discomfort and have to get up repeatedly at night. He may have dreams of being fed, or of being a child who is given candy and ice cream by an adult.

6. *Repression, amnesia, inhibition* – *Repression* is the exclusion of painful and unpleasant material from consciousness and from motor expression, particularly that part of a conflict situation which is most unacceptable to the person. *Amnesia* means loss of memory, and refers to

total experiences. In *inhibition,* the individual refrains, consciously or unconsciously, from a threatening activity. In *suppression,* the individual consciously forces an unacceptable idea out of his mind successfully for a period of time.

7. *Avoidance of the situation* – The unconscious psychological formula here is: "If I avoid the dangerous situation, I will escape pain and catastrophe." Thus a patient may have to take a train to visit someone whom he dreads encountering because he expects humiliation, dominated and injury, but whom he feels obliged to visit. He develops anxiety attacks while riding in the train, and is unable to continue the trip. In this way he avoids the situation which he really dreads (phobia). Similarly, some individuals may avoid contact with people who are superior to them in any significant way. Others may avoid situations of responsibility or those in which they have to lead because these situations are fraught with fear for them. In other situations they feel safe. Physical illness may serve this same purpose of avoidance or escape.

8. *Emotional detachment* – "I do not have any emotions which would lead to danger. I maintain my distance, my isolation from events that can cause trouble." In some individuals such emotional coolness is a constant trait; they never get enthusiastic about anything, never get really close to anyone emotionally. Others show this detachment only in certain situations; they may be intensely emotional about their work or about certain hobbies, but remain emotionally aloof from people.

9. *Reaction formation* is a defense mechanism characterized by activity precisely opposite in trend to that of the underlying impulses, or by the development of conscious

socialized trends which continue to persist in the unconscious. *Examples:* The orderliness, cleanliness of the anal character as opposed to the unconscious infantile excretory interests. Many sublimations represent a reaction formation: Collecting, saving, punctuality. (*Sublimition* is a method whereby primitive desires and impulses obtain an outlet in modified form in socially approved activities, as expressed in hobbies, choice of vocation, etc.)

10. *Rigid regulations* – The formula is: "I can guard against unexpected danger, I can carry out my desires, cope with the situation, and still feel safe only if I follow rigid rules in my behavior."

The simplest examples of this behavior device are furnished by patients who extol and insist on, or anxiously follow, a very rigid routine in work. The patient who feels insecure in social contact follows a system in meeting people. He may be able to meet them only professionally; hence he invites people to his house only with the idea of professional contact. This motivation may be strikingly present in every contact he makes. Similar reactions are seen in patients who must have their desk arranged in a certain inflexible order, or whose eating habits are rigidly set, or who consider social behavior customs of the utmost importance. Some obsessional attitudes belong in this category. For example, one patient had an obsessional fear of infection. He could have sexual relations with his wife only if she took a shower, scrubbed herself with a brush, dressed completely in white, covered her hands feet and head, and did not brush against anything--even a chair--on the way to their room.

11. *Limitation of the situation* – The formula is: "If I put certain restrictions on the situation or on the act, I

eliminate the dangerous aspects." For example, a woman patient who keeps some of her clothes on while having sexual relations says that in this way she does not give herself fully to the man. Her guilt feelings and also his domination are thus lessened. A girl who is stringly attracted to men may see them only infrequently.

12. *Compromise formation* – The unconscious formula is: "If I strive for the goal in a straightforward manner, I shall not be strong enough to reach it, or dangers will prevent me from reaching it; but if I do not try to reach the goal fully or if I use qualifications which partly deny it, I may attain approximately what I would like to get." It is also a technique of attaining both goals where there is conflict between them.

Another form of compromise is manifest when some act is done in such a manner that it falls short of its assumed purpose. For instance, a patient gave her antagonistic in-laws a present which suited her own house but not theirs. Thus she did what was expected of her, but they secured no pleasure from it.

The term "compromise formation" is often used in another sense. For example, the patient's symptoms may satisfy both the tabooed desire as well as his sense of guilt. Obsessive thoughts, in a sense, are of this nature. Through them the patient expresses hostility or sexual impulses, but at the same time he suffers. It is as if it were permissible to express a "bad" impulse, if only one "paid" for it. Many bodily symptoms have aspects which satisfy the patient's opposite urges and needs. Thus an uncontrollable contraction of the muscles of the arm may express an urge to attack, but with simultaneous incapacity and suffering.

Some patients unconsciously do not dare to take the initiative and to commit themselves fully to any action for fear of failure and catastrophic humiliation. They, therefore, maneuver so that another individual will persuade them to take a certain course of action, whereupon emotional responsibility falls on the other person.

13. Dependence, desire for complete care – The formula here is: "If I have the complete help of another stronger individual I shall be safe and I can obtain my goal." This attitude may be expressed in fantasies in which the patient finds a superior person who showers favors on him and thus makes him well and happy. It may show itself in the patient's daily behavior, as when he asks someone else's advice and follows blindly on every occasion. It may show itself in such dramatic symptoms as "astasis-abasia", in which, in spite of having no serious organic ailment, the patient is unable to stand or walk and must therefore remain in bed and be taken care of. It is manifested in some patients who feel completely lost when alone. They suffer severe states of anxiety accompanied by violent bodily symptoms, such as gasping and pain around the heart; and their symptoms lessen or disappear only if someone who is devoted to them is present. Similar conditions may be present in emotional depression, or when a patient is terror-stricken at crossing the street unless a certain individual goes with him. Investigation shows that such patients desire unqualified affection, interest, and care from another individual (Horney). These dependence devices may also be used as mechanisms for domination (Adler).

14. *Submission, obedience, ingratiation* – "If I obey a stronger individual, I'll have his protection and will en-

able myself to reach necessary goals." Such a formula in its simplest form leads to obliging behavior; the patient complies with everyone's request and is extremely humble. He may express this attitude in fantasies in which he is used, sexually or otherwise, by other people. In a woman, this attitude may express itself in her need of feeling of obligation to submit sexually to any man who pays some attention to her, even though she herself does not desire him. It may express itself in homosexual submission.

15. *Self-debasement* – "I want to submit, I want to show that I am insignificant and worthless, in order to obtain what I am asking for." Such an unconscious formula may result in a strong tendency to self-abasement, a tendency which has another aspect, namely: "I want to show him that I am worthless, that I am insignificant, that I am contemptible, so that he will forgive me for being hostile toward him, and will help me." The manifestations of this attitude can be seen in severe depression, in which the patient accuses himself of all sorts of crimes which he has not committed; he is a sinner who does not deserve to live, and he is being punished (delusion of sin and guilt). Such symptoms may, in some cases, represent not so much a purposeful coping with the problem as discouragement.

16. *Turning against oneself* – In this reaction the patient directs toward himself an impulse that was first directed toward someone else. The unconscious formula is: "I will hurt myself instead of hurting him. If I do this, I will be forgiven and helped; I will escape worse punishment." The impulse more frequently involved is a hostile one. In emotional depression the patient usually accuses himself of acts and impulses for which he really blames

someone else. The very fact of suffering and incapacity has the implication of the patient's harming himself instead of someone who disappointed him or treated him unfairly, but on whom he feels absolutely dependent. In other cases, it may represent extreme discouragement and low self-esteem.

17. *Attack, violence, hostility, and projection* (defensive hostility) The formula here is: "I am in danger in various situations, but I shall be safe and able to carry out my goals if I successfully attack and incapacitate my adversary." This device may show itself in constantly overbearing and dominating behavior, or in elaborate fantasies of destruction.

18. *Need to control, to be superior, to dominate* – The formula is: "If I can secude him (or her), I shall have mastered him (or her)." In still other cases a patient will enter only those situations and relationships, either work or social, in which he can be superior and cominate.

19. *Renouncing control* – This is present in connection with violent, obscene, obsessional thoughts. Thus a patient has thoughts of injuring others; but the thoughts appear in a form which enable him to say, "These are not my thoughts, they come to me from without, I am not responsible for them". It should be mentioned that these violent impulses are themselves a reaction t catastrophic anticipation. However, the patient's lack of control" over this or other symptoms is further "willed" (unconsciously) by him; he is motivated by fear of catastrophic consequences if he acknowledges them as his own.

20. *Self aggrandizement* – The formula is: "I am unique, I am remarkable, I possess exceptional qualities, I do not have to feel worthless and helpless. Being

remarkable gives me satisfaction, and I can also achieve other goals." This attitude is sometimes evident only if considered psychological study of the patient is made. It may show itself in thoughts of greatness, which are at times entirely fantastic, such as flying in an airplane over the nation's capital and controlling by means of death rays everything that goes on in the country. The attitude may express itself rather dramatically in the delusion of grandeur. A less obvious expression is seen in people who consider themselves superior in some respect to everyone they know.

21. *Elation with denial* – The formula underlying this device is: "I will not acknowledge my fears, my conflict, my self-contempt, my feelings of being dissapproved; I will evaluate myself highly, I will be very active, I will be happy." The patient is emotionally elated and very active; his thoughts flit from one subject to another (Manic reaction). The same phenomenon is observable, in a less intesne form, in the slighter, more fleeting elation of people who constantly swing from emotional depression and pessimism to emotional elation and glowing optimism and high self-evaluation.

22. *Failure of an organ to function in the active situation* (conversion) The unconscious psychological formula is: "I cannot avoid the dangerous situation, but I can protect myself against catastrophe if I fail." The most important organ which will be used by the patient in an active situation fails. Examples are impotence in man, frigidity in woman, headache, loss of appetite, spasm or paralysis of certain muscles--e.g., the arm muscles of a musician who dreads exposure and humiliating failure before an audience.

23. *Gratification of bodily urges as source of solace and strength*--The formula here is: "I will eat, I will have sexual relations (or urinate or move my bowels or take a bath), and then I won't feel alone, I won't feel helpless and weak; on the contrary, I will drive pleasure, I will feel stronger and be safe." The most frequent function used for this purpose is eating, particularly eating sweets. Thus, whenever a patient experiences a disappointment or feels depressed and lonely, he may indulge in food.

24. *Counteracting* (doing and undoing) – The term "doing and undoing" more frequently refers to patients with obsessional thoughts. In them, the thought of killing or an obscene thought is followed by a pious act which serves the purpose of undoing the effect of the thought. This type of device, however, does not serve the purpose of carrying out a function and reaching a goal, it is only ameliorative.

25. *Violence and self-injury* (sadism and masochism). – The formula is: "I carry out the activity if I violently attack the individual of whom I am afraid." In other instances it is: "Only if I let him hurt me or if I hurt myself can I derive pleasure from the activity." Here belong sadism and masochism in genital activity. The individual can obtain pleasure only, in the case of sadism, if he hurts his partner, or, in the case of masochism, if he is hurt. In the extreme form such attitudes may lead to "lust murders".

26. *Symbolization* – An unconscious process built up on associations and similarities whereby one object comes to represent or stand for (symbolize) another object through some part, quality or aspect which the two have in common. (Differentiated from conscious symboliza-

tion which is equally widespread; The fraternity pin, the diamond ring, language). Examples occur in dreams, literature, mythology, fairy tales, art. Not more than 100 objects are symbolized, but thousands of symbols are used (Father is represented by king, God, director, executive; the body by house, the phallus by any pointed object, spire, dagger, gun. The food symbolizes speed, power, foundation, fecundity, etc.).

27. *Identification* – An individual takes on the attributes of another, as in hero-worship the identification of the husband with the wife in labor; in delusions of being Napoleon, Jesus, etc.; the physician identifying with his patient, etc.

28. *Isolation* (on No. 8) – The emotional charge is separated from the memory of a painful impression or experience; the memory thus appears to be colorless and unimportant. This occurs most commonly in obsessional neuroses.

29. *Idealization* – The inability to see one's own faults; the sexual overestimating occurring when one is in love; the overestimation of a love-object as a compensatory measure for hostility toward the object; self-love for narcissism.

30. *Misinterpretation* – Not recognizing hostile impulses in others directed at oneself, and instead attributing benevolent attitudes to others.

31. *Introjection* – The incorporation of the affect, the wishes, the prohibitions, or the ideals of another person or person, thus representing a method of gaining possession of the other person. "I love you so much I could eat you up." The hallucinations of an internal voice in

schizophrenia represent the dissociation of an introjected object from the conscious life.

32. *Condensation* – Several ideas or images are telescoped into a single word phrase, symbol, or image, for the sake of psychic economy, and to obscure the underlying meaning. Examples: Slips of tongue, dreams, schozophrenic word salads, conversion symptoms.

33. *Denial* – Negation of reality in fantasy, in work, or in act. Examples: The boy is sent to an institution because of his mother's death but continues to write to her and to talk of visiting her.

34. *Identification with the aggressor* – After a visit to the dentist, the little boy continues to "play dentist" for several weeks.

Chapter 5
EXAMINATION OF NON-COOPERATIVE OR STUPOROUS PATIENTS

The difficulty of getting information from non-cooperative patients should not discourage the physician from making and recording certain observations. These may be of great importance in the study of various types of cases and give valuable data for the interpretation of different clinical reactions. It is hardly necessary to say that the time to study negativistic reactions is during the period of negativism, the time to study a stupor is during the stuporous phase. To wait for the clinical picture to change or for the patient to become more accessible is often to miss an opportunity and leave a serious gap in the clinical observation. Obviously it is necessary in the examination of such cases to adopt some other plan than that used in making the usual mental status. The following guide was devised to cover in a systematic way the most important points for purposes of clinical differentiation.

I. GENERAL REACTION AND POSTURE:

(a) Attitude voluntary or passive.

(b) Voluntary postures comfortable, natural, constrained or awkward.

(c) What does the patient do if placed in awkward or uncomfortable positions.

(d) Behavior toward physicians and nurses; resistive, evasive, irritable, apathetic, compliant.

(e) Spontaneous acts: any occasional show of playfulness, mischievousness or assaultiveness. Defense movements when interfered with or when pricked with pin. Eating and dressing. Attention to bowels and bladder. Do the movements show only initial retardation or consistent slowness throughout?

(f) To what extent does the attitude change? Is the behavior constant or variable from day to day? Do any special occurrences influence the condition?

II. FACIAL EXPRESSION:

Alert, attentive, placid, vacant, stolid, sulky, scowling, averse, perplexed, distressed.

Any play of facial expression or signs of emotion: tears, smiles, flushing, perspiration. On what occasion?

III. EYES:

Open or closed. If closed, resist having lid raised.

Movements of eyes: absent or obtained on request; give attention and follow the examiner or moving objects; or show only fixed gazing, furtive glances or evasion. Rolling of eyeballs upward.

Size and play of pupils (hippus?)

Blinking, flickering, or tremor of lids.

Reaction to sudden approach or threat to stick pin in eye.

Sensory reaction of pupils (dilatation from painful stimuli or irritation skin of neck).

Corneal irritability (with or without appearance of tears.)

IV. REACTION TO WHAT IS SAID OR DONE:

Commands: show tongue, move limbs, grasp with hand (clinging, clutching, etc.)

Motions slow or sudden.

Reaction to pin pricks.

Automatic obedience: Tell the patient to protrude the tongue to have pin stuck into it.

Echopraxia: imitation of actions of others.

V. MUSCULAR REACTIONS:

Test for rigidity: muscles relaxed or tense when limbs or body is moved. Catalepsy, cerea flexibilities. Negativism shown by movements in opposite direction or springy or cog-wheel resistance.

Test head and neck by movements forward and backward and to side. Test also the jaw, shoulders, elbow, fingers and the lower extremities.

Does distraction or command influence the reactions?

Closing of mouth, protrusion of lips (schnauzkrampf).

Holding of saliva, drooling.

Sphincters: retention or urine and bowels, soiling and wetting.

VI. EMOTIONAL RESPONSIVENESS:

Is feeling shown when talked to of family or children? Or when sensitive points in history are mentioned or when visitors come?

Note whether or not acceleration of respiration or pulse occurs; also look for flushing, perspirations, tears, in eyes, etc.

Do jokes elicit any response?

Effect of unexpected stimuli (clap hands, flash of electric light).

VII. SPEECH:

Any apparent effort to talk, lip movements, whispers, movements of head.

Note exact utterances with accompanying emotional reaction (may indicate hallucinations).

VIII. WRITING:

Offer paper and pencil. Irresponsive or partially stuporous patients will often write when they fail to talk.

IX. SOMATIC REACTIONS:

(a) Temperature, pulse, respirations.

(b) Blood pressure.

(c) Vasomotor reactions: skin warm, cool or greasy; cyanosis, flushing, dermatographia.

(d) Skin reflexes.

Chapter 6
Mental Deficiency

Years ago, when the majority of the people lived a rather simple life in a limited environment and performed tasks requiring no high degree of skill, the standard for determining mental competency was naturally much lower with the net result that only the more marked degree of mental deficiency was recognized. Because of the relativeness of the terms, as one would expect, mental deficiency constitutes a much larger and more conspicuous social problem today than ever before.

There is no doubt that idiots and imbeciles have been recognized since the early dates of our civilization. For the Spartan, idiocy presented a real social problem and one which they dealt with in the sternest fashion. The defective children of that era are reported to have been "cast into the rivers or left to perish on the mountain side."

The early work with the mental defectives in this country was materially aided by the personal presence of Sequin, the "Apostle of the Idiots." Sequin was the first great teacher and leader in the field of mental deficiency.

All the early schools for the mentally defective were organized in the hope of overcoming, if not entirely curing, idiocy so that the individual could be returned to his community. The early schools, therefore, were essentially educational institutions.

Although the early promises of Sequin's work were not fulfilled and the application of his method did not succeed in curing a single case of true mental deficiency, nevertheless, this method of motor-sensory training forms the basis of our present approach to the training of normal kindergarten children. Thus, the 19th Century witnessed a promising beginning of organized scientific work in behalf of the mentally deficient. It saw the development of a sound educational procedure. It brought to defeat the theory that mental deficiency could be cured. It marked the development of state institutions and, above all, it secured recognition of the social responsibility for dealing with this problem.

Mental deficiency, although it may result from disease, is a condition and not a disease. This condition is a state of mental or social incompetence implying that the individual is unable to manage himself or his affairs. This state of incompetence is attributed to low intelligence. Intelligence has, for a variety of reasons, become arrested in its development. Although there is no known cure for mental deficiency this condition can for the educable grades of persons, be greatly alleviated through planned training programs. Through the clinical appraisals of the limitations and capabilities of these individuals, training can be so geared and planned as to bring out the best in those persons for maximum social usefulness. The number of such individuals that can be successfully trained and returned to society on a full or partially self-supporting basis depends upon the severity of the condition, their level of social maturity and personnel and facilities available for training. With the scientific approach to the study of mental deficiency, many more of these individuals will become assets to the institution and their communities.

The Wisconsin State Department of Public Welfare, through its Board of Public Welfare, has general supervision and direction over the Colonies and Training Schools. Immediate supervision is vested in the Division of Mental Hygiene, under the able direction of Dr. Leslie Osborn.

The Southern Wisconsin Colony, located at Union Grove and the Northern Wisconsin Colony, located at Chippewa Falls, were created to provide custody, care and treatment and training for mentally deficient and/or epileptic persons, committed to it by the various courts of the state.

No state attempts to provide accommodations in institutions for all its mental defectives, in states making the best provisions there are accommodations for about 10% of the probable number of mental defectives. Since it is impossible to place all in institutions, it is necessary to select carefully the cases for whom institutional care is required. Social consideration rather than degree of defect should determine selection for institutions. With many exceptions the children most in need of institutional care are the following:

1. The anti-social or seriously maladjusted, i.e., those who tend to delinquency and are a danger to themselves or others

2. Those who are without homes or who are not given proper care in their homes.

3. Those who require an excessive share of the mother's time and strength.

4. Those of educable or trainable grades living in communities.

Oftenest proposed but usually least in need of institutional care, is the low grade child. He is not likely to make trouble in the community and cannot for the most part, profit by special training. He may, however, be a serious burden at home, and if so something is gained by placing him in an institution.

The physical care and training program at is, of necessity, a diversified one. Some of the children who are severely retarded require intimate care for their daily basic needs. Others of less severe handicaps are able to respond to training in self-help and simple maintenance work assignments. The more capable individuals receive not only this training, but are also given assignments that require a higher degree of self-direction or responsibility; all require, however, some supervision.

The term "training school" is interpreted to mean that every individual included therein should have the opportunity to gain new experiences and to grow and develop to the limits of his abilities.

With this as the basic philosophy, a training program has been organized at the Southern Wisconsin Colony and Training School to reach as many of the children as possible with the personnel and facilities available. The training program is divided into a number of areas all of which are closely related to each other. The training school proper is divided into three departments; the school department, the occupational therapy department, and the recreation department.

The school department at present consists of a school principal and seven teachers, all trained in teaching mentally handicapped children. Classes are conducted on a co-educational basis and are held in substandard basement classrooms. Nursery school, kindergarten, primary, intermediate, and advanced academic classes are held daily with physical education, manual arts, home-making and adult classes meeting at scheduled periods. By combining these activities with occupational therapy, many of the children receive a full day program of training.

Recent efforts of the school department have been directed towards developing a curriculum for the non-academic child whom we shall call "trainable" as distinguished from the academically educable child. The objectives of the curriculum for the trainable child are to teach the child to care for his daily physical needs, to teach the children to live with one another and with adults, to develop the child's capacities to the fullest so that he can more adequately carry on activities in his limited environment and to teach the child to play and be happy.

A second area of the school program is designed to provide a form of vocational or occupational training for those who may some day return to a useful place in society and for those who will find their permanent home in the institution. The areas for the girls include the bakery, employee dining room, kitchens, laundry, sewing room and the hospital; and for the boys, the warehouse, farm ground detail, electrical repairs, painting, carpentry, shoe repair, and butcher shop. In each of these areas one or more of the regular employees serve as the training instructor.

Each teacher of the school department, in addition to their regular classes, devotes one night per week to some group activity. The classes organized for evening school are academic, homemaking, and manual training. A group of boys and girls participate in square dancing and a library has been opened where books are loaned on a regular basis. Other activities include a leisure time club, social club, and a gymnasium program.

The second department of the training school program having four instructors is the occupational therapy department. Occupational therapy has long been recognized as an aid in achieving the final goal of social and economic independence for the slow learning child. The two units of the occupational therapy department operates five days a week. One workshop is equipped with those art and craft materials with feminine appeal and facilities are also available for weaving, leather work, typing, sewing, painting, stenciling, hooked rug making, and ceramics.

The other unit is equipped with hand tools, for crafts that appeal to men and boys. Metal work, weaving, leather, fly-tieing, wood and plaster carving, painting, ceramics, and finger painting serve to stimulate and and induce participation in a creative activity.

The recreation department, under the direction of two qualified recreational leaders, is designed to promote interest in activities for relaxation and diversion. A recently equipped "Rumpus Room" has been added to the facilities of the recreational program to promote added activities. At the present time a total of seven television sets are available, in some wards permanently and in others on part time basis. The gym is in constant use evenings and weekends. Weekly movies are shown, volley ball games are held, and square dancing groups for older patients are scheduled as well as band concerts. The present recreational program has been initiated with long range objectives in mind. Children must first be taught how to play before they are capable of imitating self-play activities. To provide recreational activities for as many of the children as much of the time as possible is a primary goal of the recreation department. Religious instructions and services are provided weekly for all patients who desire to participate in such activities.

The Statutes have conferred broad powers of transfer up on the State Department of Public Welfare. Patients may be transferred to a more appropriate institution if it is in their best interest.

There are two types of discharges from the institution. A temporary discharge may be granted by the superintendent, if in his opinion it is proper to do so. Approval by the State Department of Public Welfare is not required. In all cases of temporary discharge the patient is eligible for return to the institution without any further court proceedings. Under the temporary discharge procedure, a large number of patients are returned to their respective families each year. After a thorough investigation by the Social Service Department many, not having families, are placed in homes where they earn a small monthly salary.

The superintendent of each colony may, with the approval of the department, grant a permanent discharge to any patient who has been on temporary discharge status more than one year and has demonstrated his fitness to remain in society.

The development of a total state program for mentally deficient children is one requiring the careful consideration of all agencies concerned. If Wisconsin is to regain its former position as a leader in this field it must give serious consideration to the following:

1. The development of adequate facilities for early recognition and diagnosis.

2. Increased facilities for education and training both through state residential schools and public school classes for both the educable and trainable slow learning child.

3. Adequate institutional facilities and trained personnel.

4. The development of a foster home care program.

5. The establishment of a "half-way" house to assist children to adjust to community living.

6. Planned training of all types of personnel required.

7. Increased public and agency education to the problems of the mentally deficient child.

8. The development of facilities for vocational and occupational guidance, training and placement.

9. Adequate personnel to counsel parents and families.

10. Continued research to determine more adequately the nature of the problem and the needs of the mentally deficient child.

The aim is to provide children with the best care possible and to offer them a program of training designed to meet their physical, mental, emotional, and social needs so as to prepare them for their continued life at the school or, if released, prepare them to enter the *community at their level of achievement.*

Chapter 7
Understanding Mental Deficiency

1. INTRODUCTION.
The term "mental defect" is generally accepted as denoting intellectual defect existing from birth or from the early years of the individuals life. Difficulties arise when it is attempted to denote what is meant by emotional and especially "moral defect". Moral defect is usually applied to those cases in which antisocial conduct has existed from early age. It is generally admitted that as distinct from intellectual and emote ional abnormality, moral deficiency cannot be inborn. The term mental defect and mental deficiency apply to cases of congenital or early acquired intellectual defect as measured by methods of intelligence testing. Emotional instability, moral deficiency and moral imbecility have been classified under the term psychopathic personality.

11. MENTAL DEFICIENCY

A) *Definition* – The term mental deficiency is usually applied to persons who, since birth or early childhood have defects of the mind. There are usually also defects in motility, co-ordination, and bodily proportions. All degrees of mental deficiency are observed, from the lowly idiot who lives only a vegetative existence, to the high grade moron who is able to adjust himself, though inadequately to the intellectual and social requirements of the community.

b) *Incidence-* There are probably not less than 500,000 mental defectives in the United States including about 30,000 idiots, 100,000 imbeciles and the remainder morons.

c) *ETIOLOGY-* The mental defectives may be roughly divided into primary and secondary groups.

1. *The primary group* is by far the most common, forming at least 15% of all cases.

a.) These are best regarded as having no demonstrable etiological factors.

b.) The specific genetic background is not at present known.

c.) Heredity is not strictly applicable since only about 6% have one or the other parent to be deficient. However, all primary types seem to be genetically determined and usually show retardation from an early age.

2. *The secondary types* are those in which environment or developmental factors seem to play an important role. Include about 25% of all cases.

a.) They maybe suddivided into cases where normal development is arrested and cases where interference results in a decrease of aptitudes.

b.)   Important factors in the development of these types are--birth injuries, cerebral diseases, including congenital syphilis, mongolism, microcephaly, hydrocephalic, cretinism, pituitary syndromes, and amouratic family idiocy. It is under these titles the clinical varieties of mental defectives are recognized.

3. *Clinical types*

1. *Mongolism*

a) So called originally because of resemblance of face, skull, to Mongolism features.

Upper limit of intelligence 7 years-usually lower.

Usually good nturedlively imitative. These features more common here than in other disorders.

1. Intelligence quotient of 15 to 29.

2. Epicantic fold on either eye.

3. Fissuerd tongue.

4. Conjuncturities at time of examination.

5. Always congenital.

b) *Etiological factors*

Advanced age of mother; 50% are last born of children; possible that due to age of maternal tissues, embryo does not receive sufficient nourishment.

Birth Injury cases

Caused by indiscriminate use of forceps or prolonged labor-cerebral hemorrhage may occur in utero.

Cerebral Inflammations

Syphillis, about 10% of institutional defectives may be any level 1.q.- but usually idiocy or imbecility.

2. *Microcephaly* 1% of institutional defectives

Small head, convolutional markings are simple, brain weighs only 800-900 gms.

Ebaugh states: Usually troublesome, bad-tempered but trainable.

Henderson states: good tempered, vivacious, industrious.

3. *Hydrocephaly*

Due to blocking of ventricular outlets-swelling of cranium with a content of sometimes 2,000 cc-mental defect not sever usually.   May be caused by congenital, basal meningitis, or hemorrhage sustained at birth.

Chapter 8
CURRENT TRENDS AND DEVELOPMENTS IN PROGRAMS FOR THE MENTALLY RETARDED

HISTORICAL DEVELOPMENT

A highly developed and complex social and economic order demands a great deal of participation, specialization, and skill on the part of its citizens. Its many and varied demands upon the individual reveal a considerable number who are unable to keep pace. In contrast, years ago, when a majority of the people lived a rather simple life in a limited environment and performed task requiring no high degree of skill, the standard for determining mental competency was naturally much lower. The result was that only the more marked degrees of mental deficiency were recognized. Mental deficiency, therefore constitutes a much larger and more conspicuous social problem today. It is a problem that must be met intelligently through organized cooperative efforts on the part of all concerned with the health and welfare of all the citizens.

THE HISTORY OF PUBLIC RECOGNITION

There is little doubt that the most severely retarded have been recognize since the early days of civilization. For the Spartans, idiocy presented a real social problem with which they dealt with in the sternest fashion. The children of that era recognized as defective are reported to have been "cast into the River Eurotas or left to perish of exposure on the mountain sides." The Laws of Lycurgus countenanced the deliberate abandonment of idiots. This practice was probably followed to a certain degree throughout ancient Greece and, according to Cicero, also among the Romans.

The Greek root from which the word idiot is derived implies a person set apart or alone, thus implying that these persons lived in a world by themselves more or less outside the realm of society. It was as "extra social beings" that mental defectives were treated for centuries, with vacillating philosophies they were alternately shunned, ostracized, derided, persecuted, and neglected. They were considered to be incapable of human feelings and, therefore, undeserving of human compassion.

The example and teachings of Christ as to the duty of mankind to the weak and helpless appear to have brought some relief to the group. From that time on, there were instances of the recognition of social responsibility for the care of the mentally deficient, the weak, and the helpless. In the 4th century, St. Nicholas, the Bishop of Myra, is said to have shown particular compassion toward the mentally deficient. St. Vincent de Paul and his "Sisters of

Charity" in the 16th century gave kindly treatment to the mentally deficient along with other unfortunates whom they brought under care in the first public institution in Paris, Bicetre.

During the Middle Ages, the mentally deficient frequently earned favor and support as fools and jesters at the hands of the nobility, providing entertainment in the castles of the rich. In certain localities on the European continent, they actually received homage because of the superstitious belief that they were the "children of God." As late as the days of the Reformation, Luther and Calvin regarded mental incompetents as "filled with Satan." The American Indian on this continent allowed "the children of the Great Spirit" to go unharmed.

The first scientific attempt at educating the retarded was made at the beginning of the 19th century by Itard, a French physician who was inspired by the sensationalism of the French post revolutionary period. His philosophy was based on the premise that man had unlimited possibilities and that education and environment were the determining factors in mental development. He undertook to determine what might be the degree of intelligence and the nature of the ideas in a boy who "was deprived from birth of all education and lived entirely separated from people." While Itard's attempt to train and teach "Victor" the "Wild Boy of Aveyion" failed, he nevertheless made a significant contribution to the education of the mentally handicapped through a major emphasis upon socialization and mental training through sensory stimulation. He also attempted to create human desires and wants as well as the development of speech, with the final attempt to culminate in the development of intelligence.

It is difficult to evaluate the work of Itard, yet he clearly demonstrated that the severest form of mental defect can be improved to some degree. His real contribution, however, was not the attempt at the first scientific training of the mentally retarded. His real contribution was the inspiration he gave to Edward Seguin, known today as the "Apostle of the Idiots," the first great teacher and leader in the field of mental deficiency.

Sequin was medically oriented, and his theories of educating the retarded were based upon a neurophsiological hypothesis. Contemporary criticisms of Seguin are based upon his mechanistic approach to learning. Nevertheless, Seguin's work formed the foundation for present day concepts of learning such as:

1. Education of the whole child
2. Individualization of instruction
3. Importance of rapport between teacher and pupil
4. Physical comfort of the child during the learning situation.
5. Importance of beginning with what the child knows, wants desires and needs before proceeding with the unknown.

Seguin came to the United States about 1850. In an atmosphere of political and intellectual freedom he laid the foundation and principles which were to influence the development of institutions and special class programs. The early schools were organized in the hope of overcoming, if not curing, idiocy so that the individual could be returned to his community. They were essentially educational institutions.

Although the early promises of Seguin's work were not fulfilled, and the applications of his methods did not succeed in curing a single case of actual mental deficiency, his methods of sensory-motor training form the basis of present day approaches to the training of normal kindergarten children.

The inspiration of Itard and the combined work of Seguin and that of Froebel influenced Montessori in the area of child development. Her contribution was made in the area of the pre-school child rather than in the education of the mentally retarded. She attempted to combine home and school by duplicating many home situations in a school setting. Her major emphasis was on scientific education, and the greatest defect in her theory was the assupmtion that there was a transfer of training from didactic materials to life situations.

The 19th Century witnessed the promising beginning of organized scientific work on behalf of the mentally deficient, the development of a sound educational procedure, and the recognition that mental deficiency cannot be "cured." It marked the development of state institutions and above all, it secured recognition of the social responsibility for dealing with this problem.

The beginning of the 20th century saw the awakening to the great social and economic problems created by the mentally deficient largely through the efforts of Binet. Binet is best known for the construction of the age scale for listing intelligence, although his original premise was based on differentiating between the "average" child and the mentally retarded. The original scale was used to select mentally retarded educable children for special class training in Paris. He was interested in training mentally retarded from a social and vocational aspect so that they would not become public liabilities in a public institution.

Requirements of the intelligence tests brought to light the group now clinically described as morons or high grade defectives. The discovery that there are high grade defectives stimulated new social considerations. Surveys indicated that literally thousands were to be found among the general population. Practically no facilities were available for their social control. Institutionalization for more than a small fraction was out of the question. "What shall we do with the moron?" became the widespread concern during the early 1900's.

EARLY WORK IN THE UNITED STATES

Under the guidance of Dr. Samuel Howe, well noted for his work with the blind & mute, the first state school in the United States was opened in South Boston in 1848. This school became the Walter E. Fernald State School of today. The same year, the Syracuse State School was opened, and in 1850 the Vineland Training School, Vineland, New Jersey, was opened.

The first public school special classes were opened in Providence, R. Is. in 1896, and by 1900, several Midwest cities had special classes. The public demand for special classes influenced the Vineland Training School to become the prototype of professional training of teachers. College courses were first organized in American Colleges during World War I.

EARLY WORK IN WISCONSIN

The mentally deficient were first recognized in Wisconsin in 1867 after years of education, persistence, propaganda and disheartening efforts to secure a school of this kind. A Bill was passed in 1867 upon recommendation of Gov. Lucius Fairchild, but failure of the presiding officers to sign it before adjournment prevented it from becoming a law. After much public discussion and further delays, a bill providing for an institution was passed in 1887 only to be vetoed by the Governor. In 1891, 28 years after it was originally introduced, the bill was passed providing for Wisconsin's first institution, the Wisconsin Home for the Feebleminded, which was opened at Chippewa Falls, Wisconsin in June 1897.

In 1909 funds were made available to study suitable sites in the southern part of the state and in 1913, an appropriation was made for the purchase of a site at Union Grove, Wisconsin. Construction was begun, and in February 1919, the second State institution was opened. The legislature, in 1921, changed the names of the two schools to the Northern and Southern Wisconsin Colony and Training School.

THE MENTAL HYGIENE MOVEMENT

Most of the programs of the past and present have been associated with mental illness. Past institutions for the mentally deficient were dominated by the medical profession and many psychiatrists have become associated with the problem. Psychologists originally concerned with psychometry have more recently become concerned with behavioral adjustment in children. Public interest growing out of the mental health movement has provided stimulus for improvement of institutional and public school programs. Increased emphasis is being given today by teacher training institutions for preparation and training of special class teachers.

INFLUENCE UPON THE CURRICULUM OF THE MENTALLY RETARDED

Curriculum planning for the mentally retarded had been largely dominated until World War I by institutions and the influence of Seguin. Progressive education, as expounded by John Dewey and his followers ushered in a period of genuine excitement in education. The "activity movement" or the "project method" was used to describe a philosophy of education that was centered upon the needs of the child. Much of this philosophy was accepted by teachers of the mentally retarded, because the more formal academic approach was recognized as being inadequate.

THE SCIENTIFIC MOVEMENT

The educational Psychologist became interested in the learning process and as a result of the work of Thorndike and others, much research was directed to the problem of learning. A renewed emphasis had been placed on the three R's. Following this trend, special class curriculums placed renewed emphasis on the 3 R's along with the basic features of progressive education. More recently, educators questioned the renewed emphasis upon academic skills and attempts were made to include in the curriculum the concepts related to the personal and social needs of the individual.

There is a tendency today to direct the Special Class and even most Institutional programs of education toward one heavily laden with concepts of social living. Since the special class is closely associated with general education, its curriculum will be influenced by a social orientation.

MEDICAL RESEARCH

Medical efforts on behalf of the mentally deficient have shown some stimulating interest in disease of the brain. Some f the by-products of research in other areas has had a marked effect and influence in the medical area. Particularly noticeable results have been shown in the area of prevention. A spectacular approach to the problem of mental definciency has been efforts to increase the blood supply to the brain. At this time, however, it is too early to determine the efficacy of this type of surgical intervention. As a result of blood studies, blood incompatibility has been greatly reduced as one cause of severe mental retardation associated with the RH factor.

The significance of Rubella or measles during early months of pregnancy has been revealed as another important cause of mental retardation. Some attempts have been made also to determine the effects of improved nutrition during early infancy as a means of improving intelligence.

A tidal wave of enthusiasm swept the country when results of initial studies of glutamic acid were first reported. Subsequent studies under more exacting conditions, however, reveal that the early conclusions reached did not warrant the enthusiasm.

There has been an increase in the knowledge concerning the significance of central nervous system impairment, and much has been learned about oxygen deprivation. Venereal infection as a cause of mental retardation has been reduced by public education treatment through the use of antibiotics. The effects of excessive use of anaesthesia during childbirth are well known. The elimination of lead base paints for use on children's furniture and toys has reduced the number of mental defectives due to lead posioning. Cretinism is fast disappearing as the result of new knowledge and findings in the field of endocrinology.

PSYCHOLOGICAL RESEARCH

An increased tempo has been evidenced in psychological research directed toward the study of behavior and adjustment of mental defectives. There is an increasing knowledge and understanding of the qualitative and quantitative aspects of learning in the mental defective, how he learns what he should learn, and what might be expected of him as an adult. Newer efforts probe into his personality with definite technique, and there is noticeable effort on behalf of the education of the "brain damaged" child.

THE PARENT MOVEMENT

The most spectacular development of contemporary times has been the emergence of parent organizations on a nationwide basis. The most striking example is the National Association for Retarded Children, with a reported membership of 40,000 individuals.

Community feelings in the past regarded the mentally deficient with fright, apprehensions, doubt and misgivings. The desire of the parent groups, coupled with the mental hygiene movement, has brought the problem of mental deficiency into the public mind. The parent movement, like any movement, made requests that were beyond the ability of professional people in the field and beyond the facilities and budgetary allotments provided by legislative bodies. A more recent trend has shown the combining force of the parent groups with the professions in the field of mental deficiency.

THE FUTURE

Efforts to provide adequately for the mental defective population cannot be directed to solving the problem by focusing efforts solely upon the institutions. There is a grave need to develop a program which encompasses the major areas of the total program. This requires evaluation and planning. It reuqires the joint efforts of health, welfare, and educational agencies at the state and community level.

Noteworthy areas for consideration can be developed within the institutions, the school and the community level.

WITHIN THE INSTITUTION

1. Expansion of facilities, services and programs to meet the public demands and population increases.

2. Improved technical programs in the areas of medicine, nursing, clinical study, and education.

3. Improved standards of care and treatment for custodial and comicilliary cases.

4. Improved facilities and extended educational programs.

5. New programs to replace the need for institutional care.

a. Foster Home Care. Foster Home placement as part of the institutional social service program for those children ready for release but for various reasons should not return to their own homes or communities or have no families is becoming an increasing need.

b. Reevaluation of institutional purposes and programs.

c. Total state programming by all agencies involved in the planning for mentally deficient.

SCHOOLS

1. Expansion of special classes for all educable and trainable children who can profit from such opportunities.

2. Expansion of classes to secondary school level.

3. Expansion of classes for vocational training and vocational rehabilitation.

4. Traveling teacher to assist parents in the community who want to keep a child at home. Many parents are able to do so, but do require professional help in setting up a program within their own home.

SHELTERED WORKSHOPS

Diagnostic facilities for earlier recognition and diagnosis.

Increased attention to the problems by universities and colleges.

1. A program of continuous research to determine the nature of the problems of the mentally deficient, the capabilities, capacities and needs of this group.

2. A program for training personnel.

3. Development of new techniques for prevention of mental deficiency and new techniques for the care, treatment and training of those afflicted.

Chapter 9
THE MENTAL
MECHANISMS

There are a large number of devices by which the personality automatically protects or defends itself against threats. In general, these are reactions to crises or disturbances in inter-personal relationships. People are pushed into defensive reactions by their own unacceptable impulses, particularly sexual and hostile or destructive feelings, ideas, and urges. They arise in situations where the person's wishes and drives are incapable of fulfillment because of frustrations imposed by the person himself or by someone else on whom the person is dependent for love, approval, and security. These wishes and desires usually consist of retained infantile, pleasure-seeking needs, inappropriate to the chronological age of the person.

The aim of the defensive reactions (mental mechanisms) is to reduce anxiety tension (i.e. to diminish distress), to re-establish a façade of self-esteem, and to achieve a measure of gratification despite the imposed frustrations. The following is a list of the most common of these reactions:

1. Wit, humor clowning – The psychological formula is: "I am not distressed in this situation; I am not afraid of it; I can laugh at it." This type of behavior is used as a protection by individuals who feel extremely awkward in a situation, who find it difficult to be with other people, who are afraid of being rejected. Witty behavior may cover up their distress. They may use cynicism and wit to guard against intrusion into their private worlds which are full of trouble and worry. Clowning may be resorted to by boys who are much distressed by their feelings of being ridiculed, rejected, and humiliated because of stoutness or deformity, for example. The clowning covers up distress, but it accomplishes more: They retain contact with and obtain the affection of their friends.

2. Blaming others – The formula is: "I am not to be blamed for failure. Others around me are." The patient makes a mistake in his work because of serious emotional problems, but blames the condition under which he has to work; a man is impotent and blames the women.

3. Attempted justification – (Rationalization, self vindication) – The psychological motif in rationalization is: "I am not afraid; I am not guilty; I have no conflict because what I have done has a sensible, rational purpose." Two kinds of devices are involved here; the second is more serious than the first. The first merely attempts to make the patient's behavior appear rational so that he can escape humiliation and ridicule and self-contempt. Thus a patient may have complicated conflicts and fears about asserting himself, about having initiative, about getting close to people. He will not recognize and admit this fact, but will instead give such reasons as "It doesn't pay to strive too hard. One is safest alone. In this way I can't be taken advantage of," etc. The second type of device is seen when a patient rationalizes engaging in an activity which disturbs someone else. For example, a superior who hounds his subordinates may give the need for efficiency as the reason for his behavior; the mother who dominates and tortures her child may give her interest and love for him as the reason for her behavior.

4. *Substitution and displacement* – Substitution and displacement are very similar. Substitution usually refers to using another bodily organ instead of the one which affords feared or condemned (Usually genital) gratification. Displacement more frequently refers to emotional reactions or general activities in which the individual responds emotionally to a situation which is in reality different from the one to which he is genuinely reacting.

A severe form of substitution was shown by a married woman, who instead of retiring with her husband, derived genuine erotic pleasure from picking and grooming the skin of her back and face for hours at a time.

Any part of the body or any article of clothing may be substituted for the genital organs in this type of substitute activity. Instances of fetishism belong here, as when a person gets all his pleasure from being aroused and gratified by shoes which belong to the person he desires.

Most complicated forms of substitution are seen in the following: The individual is afraid of genuine emotional attachment, or self-assertion, or final commitment to what he wants to undertake. Whenever situations arise in which he would like to do a certain thing or in which he is requested to do it, he withdraws and masturbates or engages in elaborate fantasies of self-aggrandizement. His formula is: "This way I am safe and I get some enjoyment out of life." It is obvious that such measures are highly complex and involve the individual's image of himself, of other people, and of his activity. This device serves the further purpose of solace as well as substitute activity.

5. *Revival of earlier forms of behavior (regression)* – A good illustration of this type of phenomenon is the recurrence of enuresis (bed-wetting) in children. A child who is well trained in cleanliness may start wetting his bed again when a difficult situation arises. Such a situation is frequently the birth of another child. The older child, who previously felt secure, now feels seriously threatened in regard to the affection and love of his parents. The bed-wetting is partly a direct expression of anxiety, partly an attempt to show his need of parental attention and help, and partly an attempt to be a helpless infant and thus get all of the parent's affection. In such a situation a child may also want the bottle or the breast again.

The revival of earlier goals or of earlier modes of solution is at time equally obvious in the adult. It is manifest in some aspects of his outlook on life, in his fantasies and dreams, as one part of his reaction to situations of stress. Instead of enuresis, the adult may have bladder discomfort and have to get up repeatedly at night. He may have dreams of being fed, or of being a child who is given candy and ice cream by an adult.

6. *Repression, amnesia, inhibition* – *Repression* is the exclusion of painful and unpleasant material from consciousness and from motor expression, particularly that part of a conflict situation which is most unacceptable to the person. *Amnesia* means loss of memory, and refers to

total experiences. In *inhibition,* the individual refrains, consciously or unconsciously, from a threatening activity. In *suppression,* the individual consciously forces an unacceptable idea out of his mind successfully for a period of time.

7. *Avoidance of the situation* – The unconscious psychological formula here is: "If I avoid the dangerous situation, I will escape pain and catastrophe." Thus a patient may have to take a train to visit someone whom he dreads encountering because he expects humiliation, dominated and injury, but whom he feels obliged to visit. He develops anxiety attacks while riding in the train, and is unable to continue the trip. In this way he avoids the situation which he really dreads (phobia). Similarly, some individuals may avoid contact with people who are superior to them in any significant way. Others may avoid situations of responsibility or those in which they have to lead because these situations are fraught with fear for them. In other situations they feel safe. Physical illness may serve this same purpose of avoidance or escape.

8. *Emotional detachment* – "I do not have any emotions which would lead to danger. I maintain my distance, my isolation from events that can cause trouble." In some individuals such emotional coolness is a constant trait; they never get enthusiastic about anything, never get really close to anyone emotionally. Others show this detachment only in certain situations; they may be intensely emotional about their work or about certain hobbies, but remain emotionally aloof from people.

9. *Reaction formation* is a defense mechanism characterized by activity precisely opposite in trend to that of the underlying impulses, or by the development of conscious

socialized trends which continue to persist in the unconscious. *Examples:* The orderliness, cleanliness of the anal character as opposed to the unconscious infantile excretory interests. Many sublimations represent a reaction formation: Collecting, saving, punctuality. (*Sublimition* is a method whereby primitive desires and impulses obtain an outlet in modified form in socially approved activities, as expressed in hobbies, choice of vocation, etc.)

10. *Rigid regulations* – The formula is: "I can guard against unexpected danger, I can carry out my desires, cope with the situation, and still feel safe only if I follow rigid rules in my behavior."

The simplest examples of this behavior device are furnished by patients who extol and insist on, or anxiously follow, a very rigid routine in work. The patient who feels insecure in social contact follows a system in meeting people. He may be able to meet them only professionally; hence he invites people to his house only with the idea of professional contact. This motivation may be strikingly present in every contact he makes. Similar reactions are seen in patients who must have their desk arranged in a certain inflexible order, or whose eating habits are rigidly set, or who consider social behavior customs of the utmost importance. Some obsessional attitudes belong in this category. For example, one patient had an obsessional fear of infection. He could have sexual relations with his wife only if she took a shower, scrubbed herself with a brush, dressed completely in white, covered her hands feet and head, and did not brush against anything--even a chair--on the way to their room.

11. *Limitation of the situation* – The formula is: "If I put certain restrictions on the situation or on the act, I

eliminate the dangerous aspects." For example, a woman patient who keeps some of her clothes on while having sexual relations says that in this way she does not give herself fully to the man. Her guilt feelings and also his domination are thus lessened. A girl who is stringly attracted to men may see them only infrequently.

12. *Compromise formation* – The unconscious formula is: "If I strive for the goal in a straightforward manner, I shall not be strong enough to reach it, or dangers will prevent me from reaching it; but if I do not try to reach the goal fully or if I use qualifications which partly deny it, I may attain approximately what I would like to get." It is also a technique of attaining both goals where there is conflict between them.

Another form of compromise is manifest when some act is done in such a manner that it falls short of its assumed purpose. For instance, a patient gave her antagonistic in-laws a present which suited her own house but not theirs. Thus she did what was expected of her, but they secured no pleasure from it.

The term "compromise formation" is often used in another sense. For example, the patient's symptoms may satisfy both the tabooed desire as well as his sense of guilt. Obsessive thoughts, in a sense, are of this nature. Through them the patient expresses hostility or sexual impulses, but at the same time he suffers. It is as if it were permissible to express a "bad" impulse, if only one "paid" for it. Many bodily symptoms have aspects which satisfy the patient's opposite urges and needs. Thus an uncontrollable contraction of the muscles of the arm may express an urge to attack, but with simultaneous incapacity and suffering.

Some patients unconsciously do not dare to take the initiative and to commit themselves fully to any action for fear of failure and catastrophic humiliation. They, therefore, maneuver so that another individual will persuade them to take a certain course of action, whereupon emotional responsibility falls on the other person.

13. Dependence, desire for complete care – The formula here is: "If I have the complete help of another stronger individual I shall be safe and I can obtain my goal." This attitude may be expressed in fantasies in which the patient finds a superior person who showers favors on him and thus makes him well and happy. It may show itself in the patient's daily behavior, as when he asks someone else's advice and follows blindly on every occasion. It may show itself in such dramatic symptoms as "astasis-abasia", in which, in spite of having no serious organic ailment, the patient is unable to stand or walk and must therefore remain in bed and be taken care of. It is manifested in some patients who feel completely lost when alone. They suffer severe states of anxiety accompanied by violent bodily symptoms, such as gasping and pain around the heart; and their symptoms lessen or disappear only if someone who is devoted to them is present. Similar conditions may be present in emotional depression, or when a patient is terror-stricken at crossing the street unless a certain individual goes with him. Investigation shows that such patients desire unqualified affection, interest, and care from another individual (Horney). These dependence devices may also be used as mechanisms for domination (Adler).

14. Submission, obedience, ingratiation – "If I obey a stronger individual, I'll have his protection and will enable myself to reach necessary goals." Such a formula in its simplest form leads to obliging behavior; the patient complies with everyone's request and is extremely humble. He may express this attitude in fantasies in which he is used, sexually or otherwise, by other people. In a woman, this attitude may express itself in her need of feeling of obligation to submit sexually to any man who pays some attention to her, even though she herself does not desire him. It may express itself in homosexual submission.

15. *Self-debasement* – "I want to submit, I want to show that I am insignificant and worthless, in order to obtain what I am asking for." Such an unconscious formula may result in a strong tendency to self-abasement, a tendency which has another aspect, namely: "I want to show him that I am worthless, that I am insignificant, that I am contemptible, so that he will forgive me for being hostile toward him, and will help me." The manifestations of this attitude can be seen in severe depression, in which the patient accuses himself of all sorts of crimes which he has not committed; he is a sinner who does not deserve to live, and he is being punished (delusion of sin and guilt). Such symptoms may, in some cases, represent not so much a purposeful coping with the problem as discouragement.

16. *Turning against oneself* – In this reaction the patient directs toward himself an impulse that was first directed toward someone else. The unconscious formula is: "I will hurt myself instead of hurting him. If I do this, I will be forgiven and helped; I will escape worse punishment." The impulse more frequently involved is a hostile one. In emotional depression the patient usually accuses himself of acts and impulses for which he really blames

someone else. The very fact of suffering and incapacity has the implication of the patient's harming himself instead of someone who disappointed him or treated him unfairly, but on whom he feels absolutely dependent. In other cases, it may represent extreme discouragement and low self-esteem.

17. *Attack, violence, hostility, and projection* (defensive hostility) The formula here is: "I am in danger in various situations, but I shall be safe and able to carry out my goals if I successfully attack and incapacitate my adversary." This device may show itself in constantly overbearing and dominating behavior, or in elaborate fantasies of destruction.

18. *Need to control, to be superior, to dominate* – The formula is: "If I can secude him (or her), I shall have mastered him (or her)." In still other cases a patient will enter only those situations and relationships, either work or social, in which he can be superior and cominate.

19. *Renouncing control* – This is present in connection with violent, obscene, obsessional thoughts. Thus a patient has thoughts of injuring others; but the thoughts appear in a form which enable him to say, "These are not my thoughts, they come to me from without, I am not responsible for them". It should be mentioned that these violent impulses are themselves a reaction t catastrophic anticipation. However, the patient's lack of control" over this or other symptoms is further "willed" (unconsciously) by him; he is motivated by fear of catastrophic consequences if he acknowledges them as his own.

20. *Self aggrandizement* – The formula is: "I am unique, I am remarkable, I possess exceptional qualities, I do not have to feel worthless and helpless. Being

remarkable gives me satisfaction, and I can also achieve other goals." This attitude is sometimes evident only if considered psychological study of the patient is made. It may show itself in thoughts of greatness, which are at times entirely fantastic, such as flying in an airplane over the nation's capital and controlling by means of death rays everything that goes on in the country. The attitude may express itself rather dramatically in the delusion of grandeur. A less obvious expression is seen in people who consider themselves superior in some respect to everyone they know.

21. *Elation with denial* – The formula underlying this device is: "I will not acknowledge my fears, my conflict, my self-contempt, my feelings of being dissapproved; I will evaluate myself highly, I will be very active, I will be happy." The patient is emotionally elated and very active; his thoughts flit from one subject to another (Manic reaction). The same phenomenon is observable, in a less intesne form, in the slighter, more fleeting elation of people who constantly swing from emotional depression and pessimism to emotional elation and glowing optimism and high self-evaluation.

22. *Failure of an organ to function in the active situation* (conversion) The unconscious psychological formula is: "I cannot avoid the dangerous situation, but I can protect myself against catastrophe if I fail." The most important organ which will be used by the patient in an active situation fails. Examples are impotence in man, frigidity in woman, headache, loss of appetite, spasm or paralysis of certain muscles--e.g., the arm muscles of a musician who dreads exposure and humiliating failure before an audience.

23. *Gratification of bodily urges as source of solace and strength*--The formula here is: "I will eat, I will have sexual relations (or urinate or move my bowels or take a bath), and then I won't feel alone, I won't feel helpless and weak; on the contrary, I will drive pleasure, I will feel stronger and be safe." The most frequent function used for this purpose is eating, particularly eating sweets. Thus, whenever a patient experiences a disappointment or feels depressed and lonely, he may indulge in food.

24. *Counteracting* (doing and undoing) – The term "doing and undoing" more frequently refers to patients with obsessional thoughts. In them, the thought of killing or an obscene thought is followed by a pious act which serves the purpose of undoing the effect of the thought. This type of device, however, does not serve the purpose of carrying out a function and reaching a goal, it is only ameliorative.

25. *Violence and self-injury* (sadism and masochism). – The formula is: "I carry out the activity if I violently attach the individual of whom I am afraid." In other instances it is: "Only if I let him hurt me or if I hurt myself can I derive pleasure from the activity." Here belong sadism and masochism in genital activity. The individual can obtain pleasure only, in the case of sadism, if he hurts his partner, or, in the case of masochism, if he is hurt. In the extreme form such attitudes may lead to "lust murders".

26. *Symbolization* – An unconscious process built up on associations and similarities whereby one object comes to represent or stand for (symbolize) another object through some part, quality or aspect which the two have in common. (Differentiated from conscious symboliza-

tion which is equally widespread; The fraternity pin, the diamond ring, language). Examples occur in dreams, literature, mythology, fairy tales, art. Not more than 100 objects are symbolized, but thousands of symbols are used (Father is represented by king, God, director, executive; the body by house, the phallus by any pointed object, spire, dagger, gun. The food symbolizes speed, power, foundation, fecundity, etc.).

27. *Identification* – An individual takes on the attributes of another, as in hero-worship the identification of the husband with the wife in labor; in helusions of being Napoleon, Jesus, etc.; the physician identifying with his patient, etc.

28. *Isolation* (on No. 8) – The emotional charge is separated from the memory of a painful impression or experience; the memory thus appears to be colorless and unimportant. This occurs most commonly in obsessional neuroses.

29. *Idealization* – The inability to see one's own faults; the sexual overestimating occurring when one is in love; the overestimation of a love-object as a compensatory measure for hostility toward the object; self-love for narcissism.

30. *Misinterpretation* – Not recognizing hostile impulses in others directed at oneself, and instead attributing benevolent attitudes to others.

31. *Introjection* – The incorporation of the affect, the wishes, the prohibitions, or the ideals of another person or person, thus representing a method of gaining possession of the other person. "I love you so much I could eat you up." The hallucinations of an internal voice in

schizophrenia represent the dissociation of an introjected object from the conscious life.

32. *Condensation* – Several ideas or images are telescoped into a single word phrase, symbol, or image, for the sake of psychia economy, and to obscure the underlying meaning. Examples: Slips of tongue, dreams, schozophrenic word salads, conversion symptoms.

33. *Denial* – Negation of reality in fantasy, in work, or in act. Examples: The boy is sent to an institution because of his mother's death but continues to write to her and to talk of visiting her.

34. *Identification with the aggressor* – After a visit to the dentist, the little boy continues to "play dentist" for several weeks.

Chapter 10
EXAMINATION OF NON-COOPERATIVE OR STUPOROUS PATIENTS

The difficulty of getting information from non-cooperative patients should not discourage the physician from making and recording certain observations. These may be of great importance in the study of various types of cases and give valuable data for the interpretation of different clinical reactions. It is hardly necessary to say that the time to study negativistic reactions is during the period of negativism, the time to study a stupor is during the stuporous phase. To wait for the clinical picture to change or for the patient to become more accessible is often to miss an opportunity and leave a serious gap in the clinical observation. Obviously it is necessary in the examination of such cases to adopt some other plan than that used in making the usual mental status. The following guide was devised to cover in a systematic way the most important points for purposes of clinical differentiation.

I. GENERAL REACTION AND POSTURE:

(a) Attitude voluntary or passive.

(b) Voluntary postures comfortable, natural, constrained or awkward.

(c) What does the patient do if placed in awkward or uncomfortable positions.

(d) Behavior toward physicians and nurses; resistive, evasive, irritable, apathetic, compliant.

(e) Spontaneous acts: any occasional show of playfulness, mischievousness or assaultiveness. Defense movements when interfered with or when pricked with pin. Eating and dressing. Attention to bowels and bladder. Do the movements show only initial retardation or consistent slowness throughout?

(f) To what extent does the attitude change? Is the behavior constant or variable from day to day? Do any special occurrences influence the condition?

II. FACIAL EXPRESSION:

Alert, attentive, placid, vacant, stolid, sulky, scowling, averse, perplexed, distressed.

Any play of facial expression or signs of emotion: tears, smiles, flushing, perspiration. On what occasion?

III. EYES:

Open or closed. If closed, resist having lid raised.

Movements of eyes: absent or obtained on request; give attention and follow the examiner or moving objects; or show only fixed gazing, furtive glances or evasion. Rolling of eyeballs upward.

Size and play of pupils (hippus?)

Blinking, flickering, or tremor of lids.

Reaction to sudden approach or threat to stick pin in eye.

Sensory reaction of pupils (dilatation from painful stimuli or irritation skin of neck).

Corneal irritability (with or without appearance of tears.)

IV. REACTION TO WHAT IS SAID OR DONE:

Commands: show tongue, move limbs, grasp with hand (clinging, clutching, etc.)

Motions slow or sudden.

Reaction to pin pricks.

Automatic obedience: Tell the patient to protrude the tongue to have pin stuck into it.

Echopraxia: imitation of actions of others.

V. MUSCULAR REACTIONS:

Test for rigidity: muscles relaxed or tense when limbs or body is moved. Catalepsy, cerea flexibilities. Negativism shown by movements in opposite direction or springy or cog-wheel resistance.

Test head and neck by movements forward and backward and to side. Test also the jaw, shoulders, elbow, fingers and the lower extremities.

Does distraction or command influence the reactions?

Closing of mouth, protrusion of lips (schnauzkrampf).

Holding of saliva, drooling.

Sphincters: retention or urine and bowels, soiling and wetting.

VI. EMOTIONAL RESPONSIVENESS:

Is feeling shown when talked to of family or children? Or when sensitive points in history are mentioned or when visitors come?

Note whether or not acceleration of respiration or pulse occurs; also look for flushing, perspirations, tears, in eyes, etc.

Do jokes elicit any response?

Effect of unexpected stimuli (clap hands, flash of electric light).

VII. SPEECH:

Any apparent effort to talk, lip movements, whispers, movements of head.

Note exact utterances with accompanying emotional reaction (may indicate hallucinations).

VIII. WRITING:

Offer paper and pencil. Irresponsive or partially stuporous patients will often write when they fail to talk.

IX. SOMATIC REACTIONS:

(a) Temperature, pulse, respirations.

(b) Blood pressure.

(c) Vasomotor reactions: skin warm, cool or greasy; cyanosis, flushing, dermatographia.

(d) Skin reflexes.

Chapter 11
Neurological Exam

History

1. Observe carefully the manner, behavior, emotional attitude as neuroses frequently simulate disease.

2. Patient's story.

3. Past History – Syphilis, Epilepsy, convulsions, previous attack, trauma.

4. Important questions.

- exact date of onset
- sudden – gradual
- better, worse, intermittent, constant
- previous attacks – unconscious? convulsions?

Tongue biting, amnesia

vomiting

dizziness – vertigo

visual disturbances – diplopia

pain – sweating, swallowing, etc.

insomnia – somnolence

drugs – alcohol – tobacco

menstrual disturbances
sexual life
social adjustment
family involvement
Exam
1. Observation
Posture, physical symetry, atrophus
Gait – Terms 1. Ataxia
2. Scissors
3. Spastic
Coordination – Romberg's sign – standing
Static ataxia – finger to nose – proprioceptive cord
                    knee along shin –   "   "
adiadochokinesis – cerebellar
pointing and past point – vestibular
Skilled acts apraxia – total loss of skilled movement
aphasia – total inability to speak
Movement – tremor – rapid vibratory movement –
hand – fingers
fibrillations – slow – writing movements small made
groups
athetoses – slow irregular purposeless movements
choriec – rapid, irregular, spontan, *purposeless* any-
where
spasms –
convulsions – tonic
                    clonic
Reflexes 1. Deep – jaw jerk
biceps
triceps   -   tendon
palettar
ankle jerk (clonus)

radial   -   periosteal

2. Superficial

Palmer (fingflex

Abdominals

Cremasteric

Anal

Plantar – Babinski

3. Pathological

Babinski

O culocardiac

Muscle Strength

 - grip – etc. – equal bilat

Electrical – muscle ? nerve

Heat, touch, pain, 2 pt. discrimination

(pain supraorbital, achiles tendon anesthesias

Vibration sense

Cranial Nerves

I. Olfactory – each nostrial – odors – peppermint, cloves.

II. Optic – 1. charts, 2. color, 3. fields perimeter, 4. fundus atrophy

III. Oculomotor   Eye movements

IV. Trochlear   1. strabismus

VI. Abducens   2. nystagmus –
                          movement
                    3. pupils – RR&E &
                       react to lt. & accom.

V. Trigiminal

1. Sensation to face, eye, nose

2. Muscles of mastication – jaw, deviation of jaw

VII. Facial movements

smiling, laughing, shows teeth, forehead. tates anterior 2/3 tongue

VIII. 1. Cochlear – hearing – tinnitis, deafness, test with watch

2. Vestibutar – vertigo hot and cold to ear

IX. Glossopharyngeal

/Taste posterior 1/3 tongue – gag reflex – bitter, sweet, acid

X. Vagus – parasympathetic to viscira

Larynx – position of vocal cords, paralysis

Visceral – tachycardia, nervous stomach

XI. Sp Accessory

Shrug shoulder, turn head,

XII. Hypoglossal

Tongue – deviations, atrophies, tremors, movement.

Counterindications to Lumbar Puncture

A. Papilledema

1. Increased intercranial pressure of chronic type – tumor, hydrocephalus, block.

 - decreased below brain stem jammed into foramen magnum – resp. failure, etc.

Blood supply to brain –

Circle of Willis

Chapter 12:
Fifteen select cases of mental illness:

Case 1

This 34 year old white married female is 5 foot 5 inches tall and is rather gaunt in appearance. Her weight is 111 pounds with burns very evident on both upper arms and legs. She is wearing shorts and a blouse. The patient appears rather unkempt in her appearance and quite angry and tense facies. She had a rather worrisome frown and three distinct demarcation lines were noted there because, I am sure, of frowning all the time. Some of this may be due to her squinting because of glasses as well. some anxiety was noted. She claimed that her husband has been abusive to her and the children. She says she also has a son, age 8, who has been Autistic and severely mentally retarded. A daughter is 10 years old and the patient claims her husband has sexually abused the daughter since birth. She says "My husband has been abnormal since the girl was born." She also states "The law won't believe me, took the children away from me and they are now with my parents." She claims to have been in a base hospital at the K. I. Sawyer Air Force Base in Marquette Michigan and it may well be so because her husband retired three years ago. She has had treatment at that hospital for pneumonia, and emphysema in the past, according to her story. She goes on to relate further (Note: She drifts from one thing to another), my own parents side with my husband.

The patient tells me she has been married for twelve years. This has been going on since the children were born. "People call me paranoid only because I'm trying to defend my children." She questions having a peptic ulcer because upper and lower GI x-rays were scheduled at a hospital but it was cancelled upon her being admitted here. If needed, she could have the test done here to check further. I understand form her also that a doctor treated her for a kidney infection several weeks ago. She breaths heavily and states she has bronchitis episodes. It must also be noted that she questions emphysema, but she is a chain smoker and this may be a very important factor although these medical matters will be checked out by the consultation.

In reviewing the mental status evaluation we noted that she does quite a bit of mumbling to herself. When questions are asked she suggests that due to dryness in her throat she is unclear. It is difficult to understand her. She questions the reaction to Haldol causing this. Zantac a medication she accepts because she has had it for treatment of her ulcer before. She is glad she is getting this medication at this time.

She admits she has been at the Newberry State Hospital in the past. She said that she refused to go to counseling and so was held for three days there. This story has to be checked out further.

During the interview she did have a brief coughing spell. In view of the fact that it was so difficult to get information from her, I felt it would be important to do the Rorschach card test. I presented half of the set to her, namely, cards 10,9,7,6, and 2 selectively. It was noted that on card 9 she did not see anything. On card 6 she considered that a moth, and on card 2 a couple of dogs. On card 10 she only sees the bird and with encouragement she has rather concrete thinking, that she showed very slowed reactivity, and that she is very guarded individual which is compatible with a paranoid personality or a paranoid psychosis. It should be noted too that she admits having been to the Menominee Mental Health Clinic three years ago a few times, but apparently did not follow through. She did not realize she was in the Menominee Michigan area so she is not oriented to place or actually as to surgical history she had a T&A at age 7. She had an exploratory laparotomy at age 10.

Her past medical history shows she had a gingivitis problem, emphysema by history, and presumed gastritis with the possibility of an ulcer, hence, upper and lower G.I. tract problems. She denies any significant history of taking drugs.

She denies any significant problem with alcohol, On her OB/GYN history her doctor has her down as a gravida 2, para. 2 last menstrual period 08/09/93. This was reportedly normal.

As obtained eventually her social history shows she is the second of three children, one older brother and one younger sister. She completed a high school education. She married at the age of 23. She has two children, a daughter age 10 and a son age 8. She lived with her husband until the time of petitioning which ended up by her being brought to the hospital.

In going over some of the other matters with her I find that she had been a factory worker before she married. She does not give us accurate information so we will have to check all she tells us for further detail from sources at Newberry, Menominee Mental Health Clinic and other physicals she has seen in the past as well as the air base where she has apparently had treatment for medical reasons and perhaps psychiatric as well.

My impression is that she is a schizophrenic paranoid, manifested by paranoid delusions, concrete thinking, flat affect, with mumbling to herself episodes.

I have the impression that she is of average intelligence. The paranoid reactivity is quite severe. Antipsychotic medication will be required and hopefully will stabilize her. She is an involuntary admission. I see she was petitioned by her spouse. What information that we have been able to get from Social Service records, indicates she has been harming the male spouse, hitting him, talks to herself, she angers easily and that she has been disturbing the two children at home, one of whom is mentally retarded. She did have a 1989 psychiatric hospitalization in Marquette General Hospital as well as at Newberry. These leads will be followed up and we will see what else we can find to determine what her assets and liabilities are.

For the present, hopefully we can stabilize her on anti-psychotic medications and set up a program for her on the ward that would give her stabilization as well.

Case 2

This 62-year-old white female with a long history of chronic schizophrenia, first resided at the Pine-view Health Care Center since 1977. This recently became Rennes East Nursing Home. she was admitted to Bay Area Medical Center on June 16, 1993. She was admitted for increasingly psychotic behavior, refusal to perform her adls and inability to care for herself. However it must be noted that the Haldol medications had been decreased in the past year and this may have set off the episode. This patient unfortunately should not have vacation time from anti-psychotic medication, and if so, you can expect acute recurrence of psychotic episodes. She has been treated with many different types of medications including Thorazine, Haldol, Lithium, and others.

It is noted that she had a dislocation of the right hip at birth. She has developed Tardive Dyskinesia, secondary to neuroleptics. She has had fibrocystic breast disease and as a result has had bilateral breast biopsies done. There has been a diagnosis of idiopathic epilepsy since 1971, however she has not received any anti-seizure medication for several years and there is a question in my mind as to whether or not there has been organicity, organic brain changes or whether this could be also due to deterioration as had been seen in long term schizophrenics. She does have psoriasis, seborrheic dermatitis. There has been recent upper gastrointestinal bleeding which was treated conservatively and stabilized but at no time was it to be able to be determined what the etiology was. She has cardiac arrhythmia with asymptomatic pacs and Pvcs. She has had urinary tract infection which was rather recent but was treated an well-resolved. This patient has to be carefully observed for fecal impactions and hopefully this can be managed further and followed through when she is transferred back to the nursing home. She has also been noted to have arthritis with multiple chronic contractures.

In the workup here, some things to make note of-her Haldol level on 7/16 was 43. The average usually is 5-20. However in view of the large doses required to maintain her status, this should be expected and not be a great major crisis of concern. It is to be noted that the patient's appearance after stabilization on anti-psychotic medication is much improved. She has been described as more alert. She was able ambulate with increasing strength. Her lungs have stayed clear. She has a regular heart rhythm, and it is hoped that a more adequate adjustment can be made in the nursing home milieu.

Condition was considered improved when discharged.

Case 3

This 59-year-old white male with a past psychiatric history of (?) schizo-affective disorder was admitted on 07/28/93. The patient reportedly was experiencing increasing hallucinations ("they say be good…..Do not prey…do not go to church.") And feelings of depression with suicidal ideation. At the time of my evaluation today the patient states that he was not really suicidal, but "just giving up I guess." He was medically cleared in the emergency room and admitted to psychiatry.

The patient states that his first psychiatric hospitalization was approximately in 1971, shortly after he began experiencing aural hallucinations. He reportedly has been hospitalized on multiple occasions, at Brown County Hospital. At his last psychiatric hospitalization he reported as having been treated with Haldol for many years.

The patient denies any significant past history of alcohol or drug abuse. Hw admits to being a heavy smoker, smoking four packs a day for the past four years. He states that he drinks large quantities of caffeinated coffee.

The patient is the last of three children, having one older brother and one older sister. He graduated high school and attended some college classes in mechanical engineering. He was married for 13 years, and is currently divorced, and has five children from his marriage. He lives alone in an apartment and is on SSI disability secondary to his psychiatric problems.

father died in 1952, secondary to a brain tumor. Mother is alive at the age of 82 with a history of peptic ulcer disease. There is no family history of psychiatric disorders.

The patient was in the Navy for "three years, two months" attaining the rank of seaman apprentice and then an honorable discharge. He saw no combat.

The patient was very vague about his prior arrest history, first stating that he was arrested once for drinking. He declined or was unable to tell me the penalty for this charge. It is uncertain whether he has any additional arrests.

At the time of admission the patient complained of vague back and foot pains and of an occasional headache, At the time of my evaluation, he stated he was a-symptomatic.

The patient was admitted to the psychiatry ward, and psychiatry increased Haldol to 5 mg., Inderal LA, Amiloride/HCTV, and Verelan SR were continued.

At the present time, the patient states that he is hallucination free, although he still appears paranoid. It is uncertain in my opinion, that his is no longer having hallucinations.

Case 4

This 29-year-old married white male was admitted to the psychiatric unit. His wife is age 37, and they are on AFDC, as he has not been employed for the past year. They have two children, ages 3 and 1. The patient has been married for four years. He said that after he married his wife that she seemed like a boss. He built up a great deal of anger and resentment towards his wife in view of the fact that he felt too controlled during his marriage.

It must be noted, as we review his past history, the other factor that played a considerable role was the loss of his parents and older brother in a fire when he was 9 years old. It seems this is still focused very definitely in his mind. He was raised by his step-sister until he was about 21.

He went to high school, completed high school courses, and worked in a gasoline station. It would appear that his step-sister satisfied his dependency needs because she felt the need to discourage him from continuing to live with them. He was forced to a room and lived there for several years, while he worked at a gas station, and then married his wife. This was his first psychiatric admission.

It must be noted that he does have a sleep disorder known as sleep apnea. This, I understand, has been confirmed by picking up information from the evaluation completed in Green Bay.

In his mental status evaluation, the patient is able to ambulate well. His gait is normal. He sat rather comfortably in his chair. He has a whimsical smile on his face. He seems to enjoy the attention given to him in the interview. His sentences are goal directed. He denied any hallucinations or delusions. He presented no suicidal ideation at this time. He talks about attitude being a big problem, in which he suggested that not being in control of his temper is a major thing for him. He was oriented in all ways. He seemed to be functioning quite comfortably at a high school level. He has problems with things, that he cannot interpret problems at all. He is easily distracted. Basically he seems really quite immature and dependant.

He is on no medications presently, hence discharge could be accomplished without any need for prescriptions.

Case 5

This 33 year old single female, was admitted the hospital on 7/12/93 and discharged 8/2/93. Her admission was precipitated by her being depressed and suggesting suicidal ideation. She also had some panic attacks and she felt unable to continue working as a cook at the nursing home where she has been for the past 15 years. She called her therapist. Who recommended that she be admitted to the hospital.

The patient has been depressed previously, hospitalized twice, about two years ago in November of 1991. She got depressed after fighting with a nephew, became panicky and then came to the hospital for about four hours at which time she signed herself out but then ended up an another hospital where she was admitted for 42 days. She saw a psychiatrist there who placed her on Prozac, Pamelor, and Klonopin. Upon discharge she continued with medication and was referred to the mental health clinic but did not continue her therapy and medications as recommended. On Labor Day of 1992 she became depressed and she went to ST. Louis and was under the care of her first psychiatrist. Again she was placed on Buspar, Pamelor, Klonopin, and Prozac. During that time she gained a great deal of weight, was finally discharged and continued her on Lithium, Klonopin, and Pamelor. This past December she became suicidal again and this time she was treated at the mental health clinic.

On admission she was cooperative, her senses were well-directed towards the questions. She is quiet, not restless. She appeared depressed, she has been crying recently. Her appetite decreased. She has been unable to sleep well. She feels somewhat self-destructive, was afraid she might do something to herself and so decided that she better be admitted to the hospital.

she is second to the last of 5 siblings. There is a younger sister and an older sister. She was molested by her mother's sister's sons when she was nine years old and they were about 13 or 14. She found it difficult to work this into an acceptance state. She is ambivalent about eating and so she fluctuates between eating too much or not eating, then becoming balemic. She did admit to an eating disorder for most of her life. She is a high school graduate. She feels she needs security, is always afraid of failing. She has been dating someone for almost 14 years but is afraid to marry. She is very inhibited in many ways.

Discharged 8/2/1993.

On 8/4/1993. The patient came back into the office appearing very depressed. As she talked of her problems she began to tear. When asked why she covered up her real feelings prior to leaving the hospital on 8/2/93, she stated "I wanted to go home for my mom's birthday." When I questioned her her leaving Monday, with so many medications on hand to take, she told me that she had taken many pills since November of 1991. To me that suggest the onset of a major depression. I would seem that actually somewhere within the vicinity of 24 hour, that hospitalization became necessary again. However, I felt the need to dictate the situation in detail in order to cover the entire situation for her.

In this interview now, she confesses feeling guilty to not telling me how she felt and was aware that aware that her leaving on 8/2/93 as being perhaps to soon. She also related that she has no interest in anything, nothing to live for. She lives with her parents. She indicated she had a very close relationship with her mother and so tried not to kill herself because as she said "if I killed myself, mother told me she couldn't take it. Dad's okay as she put it, but mom an I are real close." As the patient had questioned the use of ECT I asked what her parent's attitude was. She advised me that her mother didn't like the idea of her ECT (electro shock therapy).

As she puts it "this isn't life, I feel like I have an empty body and I don't exist. I feel hopeless, I hate myself, I cry an cry. I go to sleep to escape. The voices tell me to hurt myself and my family, and I don't believe in God, that I'm ugly." When I asked who these voices were she indicated that there are three males and one female. The female's name if Jane and the two male's are named Isaac and John, abut the head man as she calls him, has no name. She also states they laugh at her. She says that Jane laughs at me because Jane is someone strong, thin, pretty, and knows what she wants, all these things I can't do and am not." She told me about an episode in which one night the head male as she puts it, came to her bed and he was angry at her because she got out of bed to get a sleeping pill in order to break away from this. This head male told her that he would make her suffer, and dropped rats on her bed, she told someone on the ward, about this and he described it as a visual hallucination to her which she then repeated to me.

As I reviewed the total picture, I feel that she is suffering from an major Depressive Episode as she is depressed everyday. She has no interest in anything, there has bee an weight gain, so she hates herself for it. She has a great deal of insomnia problems so she does require it seems from time to time, sleeping pills. She has a loss of energy, feelings of listlessness, and there has been suicidal ideation as well as attempts. Last but not least, she has also had auditory and visual hallucinations.

Treatment Program has now been setup beginning with the basic minimum medication with follow-up daily. We will see whether or not ECT may still be needed. It would seem that after all this period of time and medication and psychiatric care, that it may be a necessary thing, but we shall defer such judgement until a later date.

Case 6

This 24 year old white female who was admitted to this unit on a voluntary basis, because she felt the need for it. She was advised b her private counselor, to come here for anti-depressant medication because of her markedly severe depression which has been ongoing for approximately the past month. She states "I'm here because I believe I need help to get over my depression." She noted that she has been seeing a private counselor for the past year on a weekly basis.

She presents herself as being depressed for at least the past month. She indicated that she cries for no reason and that her entire life has been up and down since the age of 15 or 16. She has had suicidal thoughts as well as suicidal attempts in the past. At the age of 15 she overdosed with Percocet and alcohol and her left wrist she slit with a razor blade in 1991. There are still three scars noted, however it is my understanding that no suturing was required at that time so they were not deep cuts. The unfortunate thing is that she also has a background history of abuse of alcohol, marijuana, and cocaine for approximately a three year period, particularly during the age of 18 t0 21. However we must also make note of the fact that she had a previous psychiatric hospitalization in 1986 where there was an assessment made as to her psychiatric status, as well as to her alcoholic problems.

We have to make note of the fact that she is on probation presently for a felony theft. I hesitate going into it a this interview but will cover this later as she stays on the ward, to find out where this happened and what were the factors behind this situation. This may indicate that this may be the first time she has been caught for thefts, or just something that happened during an impulsive situation. This will be determined later. She emphasizes that she has not been drinking or taking drugs for the past 3 years.

In reviewing the past psychiatric history, I noted that at her stay in the hospital, in 1986 that she was diagnosed by the doctor as a manic depressive illness, bipolar type. She also had an alcohol assessment. She stated that for the most part she thought they treated her alcohol abuse because she was in an alcoholic treatment program and not too much else was considered necessary at that time. In 1991 she was on Prozac, presumably 20 mg. 2 or 3 times a day but she took herself off of the medicine. She thought the medicine made her mean. So she has been off this medication not for a number of months. I noted too that she has a dyslexia problem which was diagnosed in the fall of 1992 by a psychologist in the department of vocational rehab, the reason for that being that she was planning to go to college and so testing was required. I shall see what I find in my mental status to confirm or not, this diagnosis.

The patient has had some ovarian cysts and she is under treatment with her regular doctor. As when I look in my notes I find that the doctors evaluated her ovarian cysts they also made note of the fact that she is quite a nervous individual and felt this contributed to her total problem.

She considers her work as a janitor her recreation. She likes her job. She works for an agency who has her employed in large businesses and factories around the area.

Her working hours are 4 PM to 10 PM. As far as newspaper information is concerned she seems to concentrate mostly on comics and horoscopes and knows very little, about what is going on in the state or in the nation.

She is single. At present she has no boyfriend. As she puts it "I'm not interested in the hassle." However, in the viewing some of her background we find she has a rape history of several times in the past. This may be a factor in her attitude towards the whole general process. She does things with her son, age 4 ½, David. He was born out of wedlock. She has been taking him to the library to read books. As I understand he will be going to kindergarten next year. The patient herself has gone to a Catholic high school and graduated, but even prior to graduating she has had an ongoing alcohol problem since the age of 15. This past year she completed two semesters of social service credits. She is happy and proud to announce she had a 3.75 grade point average. Grants were available for her to do this.

She tells me she was adopted at the age of 6 months. Her adopted father died when she was 13. Her adopted mother is living and well and remarried, but the will have nothing to do with her because she is "the black sheep of the family." It seems that two brothers who are also adopted and older feel the same way. They also will not have anything to do with her.

She has a flat effect. She looks somewhat anxious. Her eye contact from time to time is rather poor. In her personal appearance, she is neat and tidy. She is alert. Her attention span seems to be a problem only in covering the details of her past few months and concentrating. Her speech is logical. Content of talk did not show any suicidal pre-occupations of this time, or even the drive toward suicide. She is depressed. She is unable to say why, however. She accepts the fact that she does need treatment. No hallucinations or delusions were elicited. Intellectual resources testing proves very conclusively that she is dyslexic. She cannot subtract unless she uses paper and pencil. In multiplication she even has a problem in doing that, even though she has told me she has tried to memorize them.

In proverbs her abstract thinking is impaired. "A stitch in time" she thinks "If you do something now you won't have to do it later." which really is a rather poor interpretation for her presumed intellectual background. She is unable to do anything with "Early to bed, early to rise makes a person healthy, wealthy, and wise." The only thing she can think of is "puts you to work."

She decided even against the advice of her roomy, Who is going on for a degree in counseling, She made the decision along with her friend, and she hopes to get anti-depressant medication to help improve her state.

She is hoping to make use of help. Apparently she has been to stay away from alcohol an drugs for the past three years. There is a problem with the fact that she might cycle because she does admit to having high and lows. It would appear from what she tells me that when she has highs she is able to pull herself along. When she is depressed she cannot get going. She just has no interest in doing anything during these points in time.

Get her involved in group therapy and activity. I will start her on anti-depressant therapy and follow along with some personal counseling that may enable her to go out and continue better adjustment.

Case 7

This 35 year-old white female, who appears older than her stated age, was admitted to the hospital because of indicating suicidal tendencies. It was arranged by the social worker from the mental health center to have her admitted.

She has been described as homeless. History from her records indicates two previous marriages and eight children. She has not been able to take care of any of her children and they all have been placed elsewhere. There is a long-term history of chronic alcohol abuse, mental retardation, and polysubstance abuse clinically. It is evident from the history that she presents that we have finally arrived at what is known clinically as an alcoholic-induced mental syndrome with mental retardation and paranoid trends.

When I saw this patient in the office initially she hunched herself up in the chair, she looked rather disheveled. Personal appearance showed extreme neglect. Her voice was sluggish. She had a flat affect. She talked about having had a hangover from which she is just recovering, as the result of drinking beer, approximately $60.00 to $100.00 from her social security check. She had moved from Kewaunee, Wisconsin to Marinette, Wisconsin, only because "there is no help there in Kewaunee and I thought I could get some help from the people in Marinette."

She indicated to me that she attended special classes in high school. As a child, she talked about her parents being deceased and being an only child. She herself talked about going to the Menominee Police Station because she wanted a place to live, As she puts it, "I've been four days on the road and no sleep, so I'm very grouchy."

When questioned further about things, as to how she felt and how she thought about things, she stated "I don't want to talk. Some people want to harm me, particularly When I am drinking." She admitted to weight loss recently of about 14 pounds. She seems completely unable to care for herself. I could not at this time get any indication of definite psychotic symptoms like delusions or hallucinations, however, it is certainly evident that her judgement is impaired. It is questionable if she knows the difference between right and wrong. She likes to say that she only gets to feel that she is picked on or that people want to hurt her when she is under the influence of alcohol only. Then she went on to talk about the fact that she does not like a lot of people around. She likes to come and go as she pleases. It is almost as though she is talking about being in and out of a borderline state of reality.

She says that she has to smoke because according to AA you cannot quit drinking and smoking at the same time. When I asked her about her AA activities, she indicated that she is only able to take 10 steps and then she fell off the wagon.

Her assets unfortunately are very limited, as she presents she cannot even write. She does need someone to look after her. I do not thing she can carry on with out a closely supervised setting. It may be that after her period of hospitalization some such group home would have to be arranged and she would have to be carefully monitored, otherwise there is no way of keeping her from continuing in the same path that she has been on all this time.

Case 8

The patient was hospitalized at ST. Michael's Hospital, Milwaukee, Wisconsin from March 12, 1969 to April 5, 1969 on the psychiatric ward. She received daily psychotherapy, and supportive drugs. Six electronic therapy treatments were needed to alleviate her acute depression; but further psychiatric care will be needed after discharge from the hospital in view of her diagnosis: Involutional Psychotic Depression with Paranoid Trends. Her "stealing" was for her, a symptom manifestation of her need to be "bad" 'as she' feels unworthy and inadequate, and she wanted to be caught and punished. There appears to be no such need to steal now.

Presently, she is being seen for outpatient office psychotherapy. She has recurrent cycles of depression, she still has guilt feelings, but these are less severe, She is on Valium 2 mg. four times a day; Tofranil 25 mg. two times a day; Premarin 0.625 mg. daily, and Chloral hydrate gr. 7 ½ for sleep as needed. She has had lifelong patterns of worry and dwelling on past errors and mistakes. This has been difficult for her to modify in psychotherapy.

Case 9

This 36-year-old white female patient is separated and the mother of two children, ages 12 and 14, both boys, who are currently living with the estranged husband, the father. She is admitted voluntarily on the recommendation of the adapt staff. She has been staying in a placement in Peshtigo, under supervision. This is the home of the patient. She believes and says to me that this lady makes her afraid. She goes on to admit, however this lady treats her nicely, but she thinks because she sees her as an authority figure this frightens her, it is just how they affect her. She goes on to tell me also that she still remembers and is upset by thinking about her father hurting her by raping her at the age of 8.

Her chief complaint at this time is that she wakes up frightened, with knots in her stomach, and that she has diarrhea after lunch and supper regularly. She also again emphasized the fear that she feels of people here. Even though these people have treated her well.

This patient has been living at a group home since approximately April 17th, 1993. She apparently had a previous episode on admission in May at BAMC facility, because there is a history of serious emotional conflict with the group home manager, as well a female resident who she felt was bossing her around. She had problems with sleeping, at that time her appetite was decreased. She felt wothless, hopelss, tired, and felt continuosly fatigued. she also had some suicidal thoughts for one evening and was admitted for stabilization. At that time she also talked about being depressed. She had trouble concentrating. At that time she was also hearing voices of a derogatory nature and was ultimately wishing that she would die, rather than to have to feel so bad. At this time, this type of depression was missing. She did have some hopelessness. It seems that this is a different type of psychiatric disorder being presented.

I have to note that even at the age of 32, she was admitted to Brown County Mental Health Center with suicidal ideation and intoxication. She was also treated in the past at the Whitney Center for alcoholism. Her first psychiatric hospitalization was at Bellin Hospital in Green Bay, and at that time she was depressed due to

Imipramine during the treatment period. She was administered Prozac and Klonopin. In six admissions prior to this seventh one. The first admission (according to the notes I have) was from 11/10/90 through 11/30/90.

She was diagnosed as having major depression with psychotic features, alcohol intoxication with-drawl. asthma as a ruling out problem, and borderline intellectual functioning. On 10/26/92 to 11/19/92, there was a question of dysthymia, but there was also a question of ruling out major depressive disorder. on the admission of 12/15/92 to 12/26/92, and 1/19/93 to 2/16/93 admissions, she was consistency diagnosed as major depression with psychotic features, asthma, and borderline intellectual functioning. On her admission of 3/17/93 to 3/30/93, she had the same diagnostic category again, that of major depression with psychotic features. At that time she received ten electro-conclusive treatments with improvements. On 5/10/93 to 5/17/93, she was again classified as having major depression with psychotic features and was reestablished on anti-psychotic medications, as well as anti-depressant drugs. Other medications to which she has been exposed are: Inderal, Symmtrel, Thorazine, and Prolixin.

There is a history of several instances of bronchitis, as well as asthma.

At the time of her admission in May, which was her last admission, she had been taking Zoloft 50 mg. AM and Mellaril 200 mg. at HS. She had been non-compliant and this may have lead to her admission at this time.

Alcohol-records indicate she began drinking at age 21. She would drink at least one day every 3-4 months, in which she would become intoxicated and then have to be admitted to the hospital intoxicated. She denies any shaking, blackouts, or seizures. She was treated for alcoholism at one treatment program. There was no head trauma or LOC at any time.

Drugs-on her own were denied.

Tobacco-She smokes about a pack of cigarettes per day since the age of 21. She had tried a nicotine patch treatment, but still continued to smoke.

Records indicate that she has a high school education with a "C" average. Married at the age of 21, to her present husband, Robert. They have been separated for more than three years. They have two children, a boy 12, and a boy 14. Both children live with their father. Both boys required placements in emotionally disturbed classes. One son has been diagnosed as having ADHD and receives Ritalin.

The patient has been living in a foster care home since 1989. Her development environment has reportedly been quite unstable and she claims that she was never allowed to express her feelings. Social history also records that her had raped her and that she showed some thoughts about confronting him about raping her. Old records, however, indicate that her father died before she could ever confront him about this situation. On the other hand, she again on one occasion said that her father was still living. I did not go into this at this time, as to whether he is living or dead. She was raised by her biological parents. She has two older brothers, two younger brothers, and a younger sister.

Her mother is living at the age of 56, with hypercholesterolemia. Father is questioned whether he is alive or dead. This can be resolved through Social services. I am not to sure it is significant at this point. Her maternal grandfather is reportedly an alcoholic and has some psychiatric history, the diagnosis is unknown.

She looks somewhat younger than her stated age. Height 5'6", weight 220 lbs., so is moderately obese. Her head seems somewhat larger than average, so it may have the factor in indicating her cretin-like features. She was somewhat disheveled when seen this date. She did not appear depressed. She is alert. She sat rather rigidly in the chair. Her gait when she came in was normal. Facial expression was that of mild anxiety. Eye contact was fair. Attention span was fair. There are no tremors or shaking noted. No manneristic or ritualistic behavior was found. She seemed to be friendly and cooperative with me. Her speech was understandable and seemed to be presented normally in volume and rate. There was no impediment in speech. Her associations were fairly logical. There was no incoherence, no flight of ideas, and no loosening of associations. The content of her talks were mostly concerned about waking up afraid, having knots in her stomach, and feeling that somehow she is being pressured to return to her husband by both the group home mother, as well as the Social service department. She feels, however that she is not ready for this. She says too that she does not believe that her husband wants this either. She denied any reference of control.

She presented no auditory hallucinations at this time. She presented no suicidal ideations at this time. She denied homicidal thoughts. She appears motivated for treatment. Her mood can be described as anxious and fearful Her affect is presently appropriate to the content. As far as cognition goes, she is oriented in all spheres. She can repeat three objects immediately and after five minutes. She can spell WORLD forwards and backwards. She is unable to do subtractions at all well, for example; buy a loaf of bread for 89 cents, give a dollar, she expects 12 cents back. When I ask her about buying pork and beans can for 67 cents, giving a dollar, she had a great deal of difficulty coming up with any kind of figure. She abstracts to similarities, was unable to abstract simple proverbs. As I understand, her intelligence is borderline with an I.Q. of 79. I am not sure where this is arrived at, but I did find this on review of the voluminous charts that she has. Her insight is impaired. She is able to equate some of the precipitants for anxiety and fear. Her judgment is partially intact as she was able to seek help. However, she finds it difficult to really cope or face conflicts and problems, both at home an in the hospital.

Although she has a high school education I suggest that it has probably been one of those liberal pass through situations because of the borderline intelligence. She is able to verbalize what she says she needs. I understand that she has worked in the past, but has not in the last number of years. She has a relationship with her husband, but I have the impression that it is minimally supportive as far as both are concerned. She is, however, in the treatment system which has been providing support for her and her husband.

I would have to describe her as a 36 year old married, but separated, female who has been in a group home for the past few years. She has decompensated and because of being taken off her medication by a psychiatrist at adapt, she reports that she has recurrence of fearfulness of the group manager, who she equates as an authority figure, as well as other authority figures she has met in the hospital framework. Old records suggest that she has been given the diagnosis of psychogenic amnesia, somataform disorder, and borderline personality disorder. She did report a spotty memory in her childhood, so I would doubt that this is all attributable to the ECT.

At this point and time I would have to say that she would have to be classified as dysthymia or depressive neurosis with anxiety features, because of the recurrent major depression with psychotic features, this should also be included under axis 1. However, we would have to add- recovered at present.

The stressors appear to be her feelings in terms of authority figures, inability to express herself adequately, and feeling that she is being pressured to go home, rather than to continue on in some group home.

She has been admitted to this inpatient unit. she was first kept on suicidal precautions for the first 24 hours. This will no longer be necessary, as she presents no suicidal ideations. She will be involved in individual, group, and milieu activity. Pharmacotherapy will be resumed. I will start with Mellaril and I will see what else is needed as we move along on a day to day basis. The patient apparently has been told about the risk benefits and side effects of the medications and understands the usual side effects, including orthostatic hypotension, tardive dyskinesia. There are no symptoms noted on admission. Discharge plan should certainly include discussion with the case manager about the possibility of changing group homes. This may be helpful for at least a short time, although I am concerned that there will be repetition of her feelings wherever she might go. It is my understanding, however, that this group manager reportedly discouraged the patient from taking her medications and if this is so, this may be a factor for removing her from the home, because she should be following the doctors directions with the manager reinforcing the need for this. Influences on her treatment need to be thoroughly evaluated with appropriate actions taken accordingly. This also includes any consulting psychiatrist which would come to adapt who may not realize the need for continued medications and if they decide that she should have vacations from anti-psychotic or anti-anxiety medications, she should certainly be followed on a weekly basis in order not to repeat her returns to this hospital. The revolving door syndrome is not a good situation, as this has been happening.

Case 10

When I saw the patient today in consultation, he refused to complete the usual social history and psychological data that is given to our patients in order to complete a full evaluation. When I asked him about this, he indicated that he had enough of these forms to complete and was not about to do the same again. He reacted generally in this type of situation in a passive-aggressive manner suggesting his tendency to take a stand and that will be it. This resistance made the evaluation more difficult. It is interesting to note that his affect was rather inappropriate when he talked about how he felt. No evidence of anxiety was noted; there were not sweaty palms or complaints or any anxiety symptoms. He spoke readily and easily of the great discomforts he felt when his muscles lock; he talked about taking pills that did not help him; he talked about going into the hospitals as he has on frequent occasions and always "I come out feeling worse then when I went it." As he put it, I can't lay in the bed and they won't let me lay on the floor and so it gets worse." In the interview situation, he had the habit pattern of sitting quite erect with his arms, crossed on his chest and presenting a rather stoic facial expression. He spoke rather readily about himself when encouraged, as follows: In respect to whether or not he had tranquilizing medications in the past, he said, "I quit them as I didn't feel I should live on them any longer. I took them from 1966 until 1968." He talked about having had back trouble for 20 years. When I tried to determine exactly what he thought precipitated this difficulty, I got a story that in 1946-shortly after he came out of the military service- he and another man were lifting a can of nuts weighting 400 lbs. while working. The other man let this can slip and the patient had to hang on as he didn't want it to fall on his foot. This, he felt, caused a severe wrench to his form which ha has never fully recovered. In discussing lifting with him further, I find however, that while in the military service just prior to this time ha had been lifting artillery shells" that usually weighted somewhere between 95 and 100 lbs. He emphasized to me too that although he had been employed for approximately 35 years, he had been sick a number of weeks each year in the past 20 years of employment. There is a suggestion that as of June 1969 there was more complete personality decompendation in terms of his ability to cope with life as he found it. He spoke about having a "Charlie Horse" type of condition in which the left hip would lock or both sides of the hips would lock so that he couldn't move. At times he had to be on the floor and he tended to laugh as he described this to me. He advised me that at the present time he has a board under his bed that makes his back feel better. He also talked about a pain going down the left leg and feeling weak and that he had this experience several times in the past few months. He spoke very easily and readily about his heart attack and cancer of the right testicle without suggesting any of the usual concern or anxiety that you would have with those conditions. This indicated to me that he has probably repressed any such anxiety to such a degree as to be converted into his present type of functional symptomalogy.

He described rather peculiar reactions to the Mylograms that he had. In 1964 he spoke about the Mylogram as causing him to have "mousey" hair. He indicated that he could not sit up for almost a week and that he had to drink a gallon of water a day before he could sit up. He believed that he had to bring up his fluid level in his spine so that he would again sit. In a general way, I reviewed the medical contents of the file sent to me and he confirmed the data.

In reviewing his patterns of living, I found that there have been influencing psychodynamic factors for many years in his life. He suggested that he has always been considered the "baby" in his family. He has two sisters – ages 65 and 69 years or age and a brother aged 62 years. He further emphasized that **he** is the only one of the siblings who has been ill _ as the rest of them have always been in good health and never have had to be treated or hospitalized. He expressed sane concern for his wife who has had no recent physical check-up herself and he feels that he has had too many. He also He also talked about his wife having had a number of miscarriages after the birth of his only child, a son who is now 29 years old and married. For health reasons, both he and his wife avoided sex for many years and now, as he puts it, we're too old anyway so it doesn't matter any more.' **From** the psychiatric standpoint, however, it must be noted that often times conversion reactions are closely associated with frustrations and disappointments tied up with the sexual life of the married person. He seemed quite resigned to his life as it now is and he told me that he has been on total Social Security Disability since January 1970.

At the present time, he reads a lot and is very interested in material. Of a religious nature that he receives from a minister in California called "Tomorrows world" He plays cards with relatives and friends; he enjoys television and radio. For the present he suggests that he is quite content with his lot in life.

It is my opinion that the anxiety reported in this patient's past medical history has not been converted to functional symptoms focusing on his back. These back symptoms have lessened his conscious anxiety; hence no subjective anxiety symptoms are found and we find that these back symptoms are symbolic of his underlying mental conflict. Such reactions meet his immediate needs and are therefore associated with more or secondary gain. He does have, as he says, Social Security Disability and he feels that he is fully intitled to the pension coming from International Harvester Co. A basic sexual conflict was suggested in the **patient in** terms of the spontaneous history obtained. He shows inappropriate lack of concern or belle indifference about the symptoms he has and this provides secondary gain by winning him sympathy or relieving him of **un**-pleasant responsibilities, It is very likely that under pressure to give up his present adjustment, he could become psychotic. Hence, it is my opinion **that** psychiatrically I must classify him as (per A.P.A. classification 300.33) Hysterical Neurosis. *Conversion* Type. Unfortunately, as this has become chronic, I do not feel that I could be of much help in alleviating hi present difficulties. Thank you very much for giving me the opportunity of seeing this very interesting patient.

Case 11

The patient presented a ruddy facial appearance; her posture was straight; and by the way she talked and sat, I was impressed by the fact that her body structure generally seemed weak and her musculature was slack.

She wore glasses and her hair was blond,

In the mental status evaluation, I am impressed by the fact that she is overtly cooperative- but at the same time, attempting to be too ingratiating. She seemed to have a need to impress me with her difficulties and how "terrible a time" she has had for many years in relationships not only to the breast surgery that she had in 1966, but also in terms of family problems and having to work to help support her second husband for many years. Although she complained of considerable hearing problems, she seemed able to hear me quite well. She sat close to me in the interview situation as she claims to have no hearing whatsoever in the left ear and some impairment in the right ear. Nonetheless, her hearing seemed quite adequate in the close situation during this interview. She seemed to feel that the hearing was lost in the right ear because of sinus trouble and in the left ear following surgery for a mastoid problem. She found it necessary during the interview to bring to my attention the prosthesis she wore on her right breast. She had cancer surgery in 1966 and this prosthesis was then given to her. From the way she talked, she is completely unaccepting of this fact, feels that she has lost something, and still, at the present time, has not adjusted to accepting this loss. She expressed unhappiness about having to live with her daughter, age 18, who is helping in her support. She indicated to me that she is separated from her husband. Because she got tired of living with him and supporting him. She described him as a person who had problems with drinking and gambling. They were married in 1951 and separated in July of this year – although not legally so. Both sheand the husband arrived here in the United States in 1952 as Latvian Emigrants. The patient had worked for four years as a nurses aid, prior to the breast surgery. General information seems to be intact. Recent and past memory does not seem to be impaired whatsoever. The patient shows a number of neurotic symptoms. These are manifested by mild hand tremors, intense preoccupation with her past surgery and difficulties, and a need for whining in order to get attention about many and multiple problems that she has had in her family relationships as well as her own body sickness and surgeries. Some emotional lability is noted in such as delusions or hallucinations. Insight, as to her problems, basically appears to be lacking. Judgment and reasoning powers generally, outside of her psycho-neurotic difficulties, do not seem to be impaired. The social history background indicates that presently she is not employed. She seems to feel that she is unable to work because of her breast surgery and continued pains in her back. She does admit to taking care of the housework and similar required task around the house. She complains, also, about occasionally being dizzy, having headaches, sleeping poorly and talks of various pains in her legs, back, hip, and abdomen. She showed me a bottle containing many Librium capsules. In review her medical files made available to me through the German Consulate General, I am impressed by the fact that she is on Dyazid for hypertension, Darvon for pain, and Cleocin for past infections. She does not admit to taking any of these medications at the present time, however, This may be due to the fact that she does not keep her appointments too regularly. I am impressed by the fact at the county out-patient clinic, she missed approximately five clinic appointments. I also understand from the review of the chart that her father died at the age of 81 years; her mother is age 83 and still living. There is a report from a doctor who records that she was hospitalized by him from September 13, 1970 Until September 16, 1970. She had these diagnosis' made: peri-menopausal bleeding; post-operative dialation and curettage and cervical biopsies; and post-operative right radical mastectomy. In the mammogram completed at the Milwaukee County Medical Complex June 13, 1974 reported no change in her remaining left breast. The X-Ray of the chest June 13, 1974 reported surgical removal of the right breast having been performed and obvious per X-Ray. The May 8, 1973 report, in the surgery out-patient department, suggests that the breast prosthesis fits adequately. Her chart also detailed the fact that she had dizziness, backache, varicose veins in both legs, mild internal hemorrhoids, and at one time, at least, had a blood pressure of 180/90 which suggests some difficulty in systolic blood pressure.

In discussing her relationship with her second husband whom she married in 1951, in Germany (later coming to the United States in 1952), I am impressed by the fact that she became quite hysteriod and emotionally labile. She teared readily and talked about his drinking and gambling. She felt that she had to leave him this past July 1975 because things were no longer tolerable. There are three children from this marriage- two sons, ages 28 and 24 years are married and away from home. She is presently living with her daughter- age 18 years. Her first husband was killed by the Russians in the war in 1946. She suggests, at this time, in view of her medical and surgical problems (but not recognizing her emotional difficulties as well) that she is unable to work at the present time. It was interesting to note that on the tuning fork evaluation as to whether or not she had nerve or bone conduction deafness in the left and right ears, that it is not possible to evaluate this. She had a hysteroid type of reaction in not having any bone reaction on the forhead or any type of response in any areas which suggests that she was just blocking-out any possible reaction psycho-logically.

Review of the psychological testing indicates considerable anxiety, multiple psycho-physical complaints without organic basis, episodes of depression, and inability to cope with stresses and stains in even an average way at the present time. She suggested that it bothered her to eat at any place other than her own home. She is afraid to be alone. She has frequent spells of dizziness and many headaches. She has often felt faint. She is overly concerned with her heart and stomach functions. She has trouble sleeping, has spells of exhaustion and fatigue, and is subject to considerable aches and pains. Without X-Ray evidence, she has convinced herself that she has had ulcers of the stomach in Germany and helped "heal" herself at that time. She does recognize that she is in poor health all the time and admits to being unhappy only occasionally.

At the present time, I would have to classify her as suffering from a neurosis, hypochondriaical type, with some hysteroid and depressant components. She is unduly preoccupied with body functions; her fears about her aches and pains persist despite reassurance. The fears, however, are not of delusional quality as they might be in psychotic depressions. There are no actual losses or distortions of function. She does not manifest either gross distortion nor gross misinterpretations of external reality nor personality disorganization. She does have some awareness that, although she is handicapped by her symptoms, the malfunctioning is not distorted. I am of the opinion that the patient was not able to make adequate adjustment and acceptance to her breast surgery. I al also of the opinion that as a result of an unhappy second marriage and the problems that go with this, considerable anxieties and tensions and insecurities were developed by the patient. She had not been able to cope with these adequately. Hence, in due time a psycho-neurotic condition developed. She is presently moderately handicapped. Impairment has to be considered moderate. The prognosis is not good because she has no insight and odes not really accept psychiatric attention. She is able to do the things required around the household, but her hearing impairment and the loss of her right breast, she would have a difficult time finding suitable employment.

Case 12

This 43--year-old white Caucasian female was admitted involuntarily on 08--03-93. She presents herself as a person of stocky build with brown hair, who is living alone. Her maiden name was Charles. She was born in Menominee. She was seen by Lynn Chevalier from the Menominee Mental Health Clinic. In interviewing the patient at the Sheriff's Department they noted the patient made such comments as 'Queen for the Almighty God." "There are children here who are rats in the occult.' They claimed the patient was under attack and that they were throwing smoke bombs on her house and terrorizing her. She considered this a terrorist's attack. She said she was screaming and yelling and this of course is in reference to the Police picking her up because she is denouncing this satanistic cult. She presented the belief that we were in the process of going through Armageddon.

In my interview with her she said that all her life she worked for God. Previously she had been a Jehovah's Witness but was not any more. She also claimed to be a queen and a king. 'I'm the judgement on earth. I have to put down satanic power." Then she went on to talk to me about Vahha being the proper name for God. She said that Jesus' name was not correct, namely J--e--s-u--s, but it should be Jasah. She said that over the years this happened to be changed in the Bible. She says she is the only one given the power to understand the Bible. She talked about a conspiracy against her. She feels the cult has been trying to take her life. She believed that she was poisoned first by a cup in the restaurant and then she actually talked also about a poison in the air in her apartment. She also claimed that she took some water into the Police Department. She gave it to a Mr. Hensley, a policemanI~Yfte was supposed to check this water out for her to find out if it was poison.--He never did. She is extremely angry as she expressed this.

In reviewing some other data about her, we have to go into the past medical history. I note that she has been on Social Security since 1985 for a mental illness. Her psychiatric history must go back that far. It is unknown to what her previous medications were, psychiatrically, but I understand that a bottle of Stelazine 2 mg tablets was found at home.

The only thing she talked about was a skin problem, probably eczema.

Her past surgical history indicates a T&A at the age of 7 and a cesarean section on 10-07-81, at Marinette General Hospital in Marinette, Wisconsin.

I would suppose we could think of it only as Stelazine because this was found at home, but I question whether it was taken on a regular basis.

There is a possible contact dermatitis to certain soaps.

Alcohol--No significant history. Drugs--She has tried marijuana in the past. but will not qo into detail. She smoked one package of cigarettes for years but quit ten years ago. She drinks about 2-4 cups of decaffeinated coffee or caffeinated coffee daily.

She is the fourth of six children. There are two older brothers and one older sister, one younger brother and one younger sister. She has a high school education and approximately one year of college studying fashion merchandising. She was previously married, but is divorced. She has one 11 –year-old son, but the son must be placed elsewhere, maybe with her ex-husband, as the patient lives alone.

Her mother is alive at the age of 80, health history is unknown. Father died at 70 of colon carcinoma. Her sister also has a previous psychiatric hospitalization.

At present she presents no physical complaints, but she is extremely disturbed that she is held, as she puts it, against her will. She is extremely agitated when this comes up.

I must say that in the psychiatric interview she presents the following features:

1. She is guarded, suspicious and delusional. She presented these religious delusions with very little encouragement. She seems to be completely preoccupied with this. When she feels that in any way this is questioned she becomes very agitated, disturbed, noisy.

2. Her intellectual resources are difficult to check at this time.

She does not cooperate too wefi to ordinary questions. She will not answer as to interpretations as presented to her on proverbs. The whole reactivity indicated that at anytime she might strike out at anybody. She cannot e reasoned with. She is completely disorganized as a schizophrenic, the apparent ideation so extreme we have to be concerned that she might harm herself or someone else. Hence, it was necessary shortly after admission to administer oral medications and I even left an order for injection. This actually became necessary in time. She had to go into the quiet room. Finally, after some period of time, she quieted down. She still maintains these delusional systems. It was necessary to give her a mixture of Haldol 5 mg and Ativan 2 mg and Benadryl 50 mg, stat, IM. A pm order was left because of undue agitation. We also started her on Haldol 5 mg tid as well as 10 my orally as necessary. Cogentin 2 mg orally or IM bid was also added. It was felt, however, that these medications may have to be stopped so she can present her paranoid ideation as the are rather than to have them too well controlled for her court hearing. All medication will be held August 10 and 11. After the August 11 court preceding then we can resume the medications.

Schizophrenia, paranoid type, with acute agitation. The prognosis is guarded. This patient will require long-term outpatient care. It is questionable as to whether she can be relied upon to take her medication regularly. An IM type of medication supervised by the Menominee County Mental Health Clinic may be necessary. It is my hope that follow-up care can be continued so repeated hospitalizations may not be necessary.

Case 13

This patient was admitted to the Bay Area Medical Center on 08/01/93. Upon her admission she presented herself as a 31-year-old white single female who was blond and slender. Appearances indicate that she has not been taking care of her personal grooming too well. She is of average height, slender. Her manner of dress was rather disheveled. Hygiene I would have to consider fair at best. She pretty well stay put in her chair, although she did shuffle around a bit, posture was somewhat s'ouched. Facial expression for the most part seemed rather neutral General body movements were such to suggest a rather inappropriate type of behavior in terms of responding. She was rather slow –in all her responses, so wou~d have to consider a psychomotor retardation problem. There were no evident signs of distress. Eye contact was poor. There was a tendency to avoid direct eye contact.

In talking to her she indicated that she still had a feeflng of a blood pressure duff being on her arm and that this was a very difficult thing for her to accept. She indicated that for some time now she has had poor sleep. She cannot settle down because she feels too tense. However, thIs is not evident superficially. She suggested to me that she had been on some Xanax medication for anxiety from a psychiatrist in Tucson, Arizona. She rambles on to also tell me that the bottle was supposed to last her forever because she was to take it as she needed it. She rambled on also to talk about crossing the street, and losing weight, and talked about not being very talented. Then she mutters further that she is not as restricted as she was. There was some loose talk about an Olaf Sherman, whom she was unsure of being her father or not. Then she went on to talk about graduating from a high school in Wisconsin.

Generally, she gives the appearance that she is really unable to care for herself. She appears definitely incompetent, is very disorganized in how she handles herself and how she handles things generally. As I review the situation, I have to say that the only way to treat this patient is by way of a commitment and so a petition has been accordingly set up in order to accomplish this. Becauseg basically, she shows these following features of a schizophrenic reaction, namely:

1. Incoherence occasionally.
2. Marked loosening of associations.
3. Flat and inappropriate affect.

4. Disorganization markedly in her behavior.

5. She seems unable to adequately to care for her own personal needs.

Her judgement generally seems to be quite impaired, as a results, because of that, she could harm herself. I would doubt that she wou~d strike out, unless someone was unduly pressuring her. Past behavior and conduct as a homeless person suggested the need for supervised treatment in a setting that would help her further. I noted that she was picked up by the Menominee Sheriffs Department. They concluded that she was disoriented and quite incoherent. So, there was some evidence to feel that she does need care and treatment as such provided by the Bay Area Unit.

Case 14

This admission occurred on 7/21/93 after evaluation a psychiatrist at the Menominee County Mental Health. He felt that this man, age 37, white male who has had chronic schizophrenia for many years, was presenting marked psychotic symptoms only because of not taking his antipsychotic medications as prescribed. Upn admission he showed confused and disturbed thinking in regard to Jesus and religion, associated with his mother's name Mary and his father's name Joseph. Navane therapy gradually increased to 25 mg at bedtime and this proved a stabilizing influence and this should be continued as long as no extrapyramidal symptoms occur. This patient had a serious medical prob~eni as well, namely unspecified hypercoagulability state requiring Couniadin therapy. Presently he is on 15 mg daily. He also received some Ativan 1 mg q 4 h pm for anxiety. This however does not seem to be needed upon discharge. His dosage upon discharge will be actually that of Navane 25 mg at bedtime and he can be further monitored by continuing his care at the Menominee Community Mental Health Clinic.

AXIS I:

1. Schizophrenia, undifferentiated, chronic. Code i~295.Y2.

2. Personality disorder, schizotyptal. Code #301.22

3. Alcohol dependence and abuse requiring two designated codes: 303.90 and 305.00.

AXIS III:

Per Dr. Skowron, consultant were as follows:

1. Unspecified hypercoagulability as well as multiple varicosities.

AXIS IV:

Minimal pscyhosocial stressors may precipitate either alcohol abuse and/or acute psychotic episodes. His present episode however occurred because of non--compliance with taking anti-psychotic medication.

AXIS V:

Upon admission, GAF was 20, upon discharge 70.

The patient is on Social Security disability and seems to be dependent on same presently.

Case 15

SUMMARY: This 34-year-old white female, with a past history of anorexia" and multiple sclerosis was admitted 07/30/93, for (?) depression with suicidal ideation. When confronted with this history, the patient stated where she ever got that, I don't know...I think she kind of jumped the gun a little bit." She was reportedly despondent about her pending divorce. Additionally, she desired help with her eating disorder. She reported that she was increasingly 'stressed" because of a 'weight gain" which resulted in her waistline increasing from 21 to 24 inches. She reports that she has increasing problems with her eating disorder when she has increased stress, then giving several examples such as #1: when her dog got sick, #2. when her grandmother died 7 years ago. #3. when her grandfather died 6 years ago.

She was admitted on July 30, 1993, with admission psychiatric diagnoses of:

1. Reactive depression.

2. Borderline personality disorder.

3. Anorexia, and a medical diagnosis of multiple sclerosis.

1. First psychiatric hospitaUzation was in Madison (University Hospital) in 1982, for a two week period.

2. Multiple hospitalizations at Bellin Psychiatric Hospital, the last being a *1* day stay during the summer of 1992.

3. Treated by her private psychiatrist, Cr. Donarski (Green Bay) for a ten year period until May of 1992. She has been foilcwed by Menominee County Community Mental Health ever since.

4. Despite stating that she has been followed by MGCMH, she states that the therapist at ADAPT, arranged her Madison hospitalization approximately 3--4 weeks ago. She was hospitalized there for a one week period.

5. Admitted to Rogers Hospital (Milwaukee area) for an eating disorder from 11/3 through 11/5/92. She was reportedJy discharged from this program secondary to non-compliance.

1. Seizure disorder at the age of 1 and 14-because "my teeth were coming I n.

2. Eating disorder. Currently has a diagnosis of anorexia (which was first diagnosed in 1982), and is on a vegetarian diet since the age of 5. She reports that she has been a vegetarian since this age, when her cousin pointed out a slab of meat in a meat market and stated that's one of our relatives." She states that her anorexia began in high school with peer pressure and Twiggy, the model, and the magazines...." She states that she wished to be more shapely and pretty like her husband's sisters, stating that she wanted to be like them." She offers that as a child "I couldn't get dirty. ..I was daddy's little girl.-

Gastritis, by history.

Multiple sclerosis, diagnosed at the age of 23. She reports that she has bad occasional numbness of the hands, of the bottoms of her feet, does not diaphorese, has had a period of amaurosis fugax of the left eye, has optic nerve problems, has bilateral (left greater than right) weakness, and bad an MRI at Bellin Hospital. She uses a straight catheter in order to void, stating that her physician told her 'everything just tenses up and it doesn't release." She uses a wheelchair for locomotion. Recent urinary tract infection, when the patient states she was given inadequate water supplies to cleanse her straight catheter during her recent Madison hospitalization.

1. 1 & A at the age of 4L
2. Tubal ligation in 1982.
3. Elective abortion, 6/7/82.

1. The patient has previously been on Prozac 'on and off' for the past four years. She has not taken this medication for several weeks.

2. Recently finished a course of penicillin last week for urinary tract infection.

Last normal period was approximately 10 years ago. She reportedly has had occasional days of spotting, approximately four in the past ten years. She reports that she resumes vaginal bleeding when her weight goes above a certain level, but is unaware of what this weight might be. She is gravida III, para II, AB I.

The patient is the eldest of two children and is a high school graduate. She was married at the age of 20 and remains married to her first husband. She has two sons, age 14 and 11. She states that her eldest son is supposed to be perfect.' She then states that she was supposed to be perfect. Contrastingly, she states that her youngest son 'thrives on dirt." He reportedly has been before the judiciary on several occasions because of delinquent behavior. She is reportedly currently in the process of divorce, being served divorce papers at the time of her hospitalization in Rogers Hospital/Milwaukee in November of 1992. She is on **SSI** and medical assistance and has lived in a foster home from November of 1992, through April of 1983.

Father has a history of insulin dependent diabetes- and a brother reportedly was previously admitted to Brown County for poor impulse control.

Divorce pending.

Arrested for shoplifting for stealing an exercise tape. She received an unspecified fine.

No significant alcohol, caffeine, or illicit drug abuse history. She reports that she smoked one pack per day of cigarettes for 18 years, stopping in December of 1992. she then admits that she smokes "on and off once in a while.-

She states that she previously abused diuretics, diet pills, and laxatives for a 3--4 year period until 7 years ago.

Patient complains of occasional numbness of the hands, numbness of the soles of her feet, states that she is easily fatigued and has poor dexterity. She states that she has poor balance and feels that she will fall over when she is standing, although this sensation is not lateralized. She states that she tolerates heat poorly.

Urine toxicology is negative. WBC is **4.2,** HGB **13.0,** and platelet count **305,000. Chem 1** panel revealed normal electrolytes **and** renal function, with normal calcium, phosphorus, and magnesium levels. LDH was 187 (94--172), AST 52 (8-42), and ALT 100 (0-55). GGT was normal at 16. Cholesterol was elevated at 247, with normal triglycerides. Serum ethanol level was 0. Syphilis serology and thyroid function testing remain pending. EKG revealed a normal' sinus bradycardia with a rate of 57, with no acute changes. Chest x-ray results are pending.

AXIS I:

1. Anorexia nervosa, by history. This appears confirmed at the present time. Definitive diagnosis is deferred to psychiatry.

2. Dr. Bowman's admission diagnoses also mentioned "reactive depression."

Will confirm psychiatric diagnoses

AXIS **II:**

1. Borderline personality disorder, as per the previous psychiatrist.

AXIS III:

1. Multiple sclerosis by history. The patient apparently currently has problems with proprioception, with

asymmetric reflexes. No other neuro-logic deficits were elicited at this time.

Tubal ligation, 1982.

PLAN:

Patient was admitted to psychiatry, and psychiatric treatment is deferred to psychiatry. I will attempt to obtain prior psychiatric records. And whichever hospital she was in in Madison recently. ADAPT will be contacted to determine the name of this hospital. I have also requested previous neurology records including MRI results. I have suggested that nursing should maintain the patient's straight catheter, catheterize her only for abdominal distention or significant abdominal discomfort, and measure the resultant urinary output. I will continue to monitor this patient's medical course during her hospitalization, and will advise should additional active axis III interventions be recommended.

Chapter 13
Learn to understand the mental illness of Depression

Depression is more than a day of feeling low. It is long-lasting, often recurring illness as real and disabling as heart disease or arthritis. Adults who experience clinical depression may feel an oppressive sense of sadness, fatigue, and guilt. Performing on the job may be difficult....going out with friends may be increasingly isolated from family and colleagues-helpless, helpless, worthless, and lost.

Depression is a very common emotional illness. It affects about 10 percent of the U.S. population or more than 17.6 million people every year. One in four women and one in 10 men will experience a depressive episode in their lifetime.

Modern research has led to significant advances. Today there are extremely effective treatment for depression. Between 80 to 90 percent of those with depression can be successfully treated. Many experience relief from symptoms within three to six weeks. Treatment is generally necessary-people with depression cannot snap out of it on their own, nor will it go away.

HOW DO YOU KNOW IF A PERSON HAS DEPRESSION?

If you or a person you know has exhibited four or more of the following symptoms for more than two weeks, professional help should be considered:

Sleeping to much or to little

Frequent wakening in the middle of the night

Eating to much or to little

Inability to function at work or school

Headaches, digestive disorders, nausea, pain with no medical basis

Excessive crying

Thoughts of death or suicide

Lack of energy, constant fatigue

Slowed thinking

Difficulty in concentrating, remembering, making decisions

Loss of interest in daily activity

Loss of sex drive

Persistent feelings of sadness, anxiety, hopelessness

Restlessness, agitation, irritability

Feelings of inappropriate guilt or worthlessness

WHAT CAUSES DEPRESSION?

We know that depression results from an interaction of several factors-environmental, biological, and genetic.

Environmental Factors. Stress resulting from the loss of a job, death of a family member, divorce, or ongoing health of family problems can trigger depression.

Biological Factors. Depression may also be tied to disturbances in the bio-chemicals that regulate mood and activity. These bio-chemicals, called neurotransmitters, are substances that carry impulses or messages between nerve cells in the brain. An imbalance in the amount or activity of neurotransmitters can cause major disruptions in thought, emotion, and behavior.

Some people develop depression as a reaction to other biological factors such as chronic pain, medications, hypothyroidism, or other medical illness.

Genetic Factors. Because depression appears to be linked to certain biological factors, people can inherit a pre-disposition to develop depression. In fact, 25 percent of those people with depression have a relative with form of this illness.

Doctors know more about depression than perhaps any other emotional illness. Because of research and medical advancements, 80 to 90 percent of those with a depressive disorder can be treated successfully.

Evaluation: a complete evaluation with a qualified professional is the first step in seeking treatment. Only a licensed physician or psychologist can diagnose a person with a psychiatric disorder. During the diagnostic evaluation, the physician or psychologist will determine if any other factors are contributing to or even causing the depressive behavior.

Professional counseling: Various psycho-therapies are commonly used in the treatment of depression focus on the cause an effects of the illness. Cognitive therapy helps patients change negative thoughts or perceptions, such as high achievers who are convinced they are failures.

Medication: Sometimes used in combination with psychotherapy, medication can correct the biochemical imbalances that may cause depressive episodes. When carefully prescribed and monitored by a physician, medications can relieve symptoms in three to six weeks.

WHO MAY BE AT RISK FOR DEPRESSION?

People who have a family member with depression.

People who have experienced a stressful or traumatic life event.

People who lack the social support of a spouse, friends, and extended family

People who abuse drugs or alcohol

People who have chronic medical illnesses or persistent pain.

IF YOU THINK YOU HAVE DEPRESSION...

Remember, your depression is not your fault and it can be effectively treated.

Seek treatment. Don't let misconceptions about emotional illness or the discouragement of your depression stop you. Either on your own, or by asking a friend or family member, contact yourfamily doctor, community mental health center, or medical office for help.

In the weeks until treatment becomes effective, you can take some simple steps to help you deal with life on a day-to-day basis: break large tasks into small steps; set easily managed priorities; participate in light exercise and relatively undemanding social activities, such as attending a movie or visiting a friend. Simply being with others can be helpful.

IF SOMEONE YOU CARE ABOUT HAS DEPRESSION...

Encourage treatment. remember that the symptoms of depression may prevent a person from trying to get help. Your personal doctor, mental health center, or local psychiatric hospital will be able to help you find a treatment specialist.

Adjust your expectations and offer support, understanding, and encouragement.

Demonstrate that you know the person is in pain.

When the person says or does something upsetting because of the depression, try to put your reaction into calm, reasonable words. This will help the person understand how his or her conduct effects others, and help you better cope with a trying situation.

DEPRESSION AND SUICIDE...

Thoughts of death and suicide are a typical symptom of depression. An estimated 15 percent of those with depression commit suicide over a lifetime, and depression is considered to be underlying cause in half of all suicides. Because depression can have fatal consequences, treatment should not be delayed. Any mention of suicide-such as "I wish I were dead," or "Everyone would be better off without me" –should be taken seriously.

THERE IS HOPE IN LEARNING MORE.

Reach out for help...because the more you learn about depression, the better you will understand that it has specific causes and effective treatments. And like any illness, depression can affect anyone at any time.

By reaching out for information you can recognize the signs and symptoms of depression. That knowledge may someday allow you to help someone to get the treatment he or she needs to live a healthy and fulfilling life.

Chapter 14
The treatment of Mentally Depressed States in the Aged

Four premises must be considered in the depression of the aged, The stress tolerance decreases with age. There is the increased number of defects that appear in functioning of the older person, e.g. memory failure, cardiac, kidney, disorganization occurs when stress reaches a critical point, and The progressive decline in the capacity to experience pleasure. Now there are a number of theories that have to do with depression itself. I would like to discuss the bio-chemical because it seems to be most prevalent now, and then later on give you some background on psychological aspects of depression. Munn and Quastel some years back demonstrated that aldehyde resulting from the action of the amine oxodose enzymes actually inhibit brain respi-rations. They do so by causing reduction of the rate of the oxygen absorption of the brain tissue. Therefore any agent, any factor that blocks or destroys these enzymes produces some therapeutic affect on depression. Now it must be noted that in the research field it has been possible to demonstrate quite conclusively that these same enzymes are vulnerable to destruction by anoxia or lack of oxygen. And there are some who feel quite strongly today that the electric shock therapy or electrotonis therapy, actually plays a part in this, because with seizures or convulsions there is an inhibition of oxygen. And then, of course, there is such literature that has to do with drugs that inhibit the enzyme monamine oxydose e.g. Marsilid, Marplan, Ultran, and Nardil.

What is a depression- a syndrome, a symptom or a non-logical entity? Many psychiatrist are still questioning its proper consideration. The depressive syndrome by definition can be discussed in terms of two groupings, primary symptoms and, secondary symptoms. This grouping will lend itself to a better understanding of what is meant by a depressive state or depressive reaction. Primary symptoms include a sad, despairing mood which presents clinically a decrease in mental productivity and reduction of drive, and a retardation or agitation in the field of expressive motor responses. In the severe or the so-called very pathological depression, we also have secondary symptoms occurring such as feelings of hopelessness, obsessive-compulsive behavior. Other secondary symptoms are ideas of self-accusation, self-depreciation, nihilistic delusions, self-destructive tendencies, paranoid delusions, and hallucinations, etc.. A patients history often reveals complaints of not sleeping to well, appetite loss, and weight loss. Review of the historical development as well, enlightens us further. As early as fourth century B.C., Hippocrates actually mentioned depression and melancholia. Aerteus, another physician of the first century A..D. noted that melancholia seemed to be a modification of mania and did not affect the intellectual facilities of the patient in any way whatsoever. It took some period of centuries, however, before Falret in 1954 published the first work on manic depressive psychosis with the terminology of la folie circular. However, the term manic depressive psychosis itself was first used by Kraepelin in 1899. Of further psychiatric interest are Freud's classical papers on mourning and melancholia of 1917. There he emphasizes that depression is a complete or partial loss of self-esteem. The depressed person tries to undo the loss but aggravates it unfortunately by pathological intro-jection of the ambivalently loved-so-object. Hence, patients indulge in self reproach and present an accusation against the person who is deceased. Abraham in 1924 did some rather fundamental research upon the dynamics of manic depressive psychosis. He stresses the pregenital foundation. He talks about patients who are ambivalent toward themselves as well as their loved objects, and, who in between their depressed states, actually indulge in oral-sadistic tendencies. Interestingly, he notes that anxiety and depression are related to each other in the same way as fear and grief.

Sociologists, in comparing societies, have noted that depressions are actually quite rare in primitive societies. There seems to be less emphasis on individual responsibilities in primitive society, but in the Greek, Hebrew, and Christian culture there is much more emphasis on individual responsibility. One may question the attainment of goals in the aged. Do they feel frustrated because they can't continue doing things they feel are important to do? Can the aged measure up to the individual responsibilities expected? These cultural factors may mean much to setting the stage for a depression.

Management of depressed states in the aged includes psycho-therapy supportively, with the main treatment being organic. The main treatment is organic, as electric therapy or a drug therapy may be necessary and psycho-therapy of depression is extremely difficult. Because in the first place it is difficult to approach the patient. There is always a suicidal danger. There is always ambivalence towards the therapist. They want help from the therapist, but at the same time they won't accept what you are trying to do for them. They often times turn against the therapist, turn against their family or manage to have their families turn against the therapist. In any event, they escape from really getting help. And lastly, but not leastly, if not in a stuporous depression, they can be very aggressive in their demands upon the therapist. So often, the only way to treat a depressed patient of any severe degree, is in the hospital. Trying to do it in the office actually means asking for difficulties and problems. As yet, there has been no acceptable dynamic formulation of depression. We are not able to predict the occurance or re-occurance of depression even persons whose psychic structure is well known and whose ego organization has been completely investigated. Not only that, but there has been some recognition among some psychiatrists that some depressions occur during psycho-therapy or analysis when under treatment to relieve other symptoms. And so one can't always determine why, nor can one predict who is going to become depressed and who is not. This holds true to some extent for other mental illness as well.

There are various kinds of depressive types. One grouping consist of these individuals who are depressed with a rather definite schizophrenic background and who are very resistive to therapy. There are depressions among the pseudo-neurotic schizophrenics. The pseudo-neurotic schizophrenics is ine who escapes facing his responsibilities by multiple types of complaints, by chronic mal-adjustment, and difficulties in close personal relationships, and ambivalence. These individuals are also quite resistant to therapy. The endogenous depressions, like the manic depressive cases, the involutionals, are amenable to therapy but even then some cases are quite refractory to both electronic therapy and drug therapy as well psychotherapy. Whenever you get a patient who shows as admixture of anxiety and more fear. With a history of phobias, obsessive-compulsive personality, or other neurotic traits, avoid electronic therapy. Reactive depressions do extremely well with electro-convulsive therapy, particularly within the first six months of therapy. Many of the milder reactive depressions do quite well nowadays with some of the anti-depressant drugs and office psycho-therapy.

Are there any particular contraindications for shock therapy? Age is not, There is no medical or surgical contraindications for electro-conclusive therapy apart from recent cardiac infarction. This is the modern attitude.

Considering anti-depressant in use, it might be worthwhile to spell out terms, because so frequently, terms are used rather loosely. Anti-depressants are psycho-activators. This is a term used by Klein in his research work and it's very appropriate. He subdivides them into, psycho-motor stimulants, such as Dexedrine, Methadrine, Desoxyn, Ritalen, and Meratran, psycho-stimulants, such as Tofraniland Deanar, andpsychic energizers such as Monamine oxydose inhibitors such as Marsilid, Nardil, Cabron, Niamid, and Marplan. Here are suggestions from clinical experience: Tofranil is a very worthwhile agent in reactive depressions and manic depressive psychosis. In psycho-neurotic cases, when there is anxiety with depression. Ritalen therapy and Dexamyl or Dexedrine are aids. Drugs such as Marsalid or Nardil do well in angina pectoris problems with neurotic symptom-tology. Cases that require corticosteroid therapy, do best with Catron. In long term neurotic cases, Niamid is a very helpful preparation in doses of 25 to 250 mg. Marplan seems to have specificity in terms of helping chronic rheumatic arthritis.

As a concluding paragraph it must be emphasized that the psycho-activators are classified under psycho-pharmaceuticals. All psychiatric drugs can be labeled psycho-pharmaceuticals. Psychiatric fall into three categories, psycho-hibitors, which include hypnotics, muscle relaxants, ataractic drugs (neuroleptics), and undetermined, psycho-activators, previously discussed, and psycho-to-mimetics, which are the research drugs for the most part, such as Lysergic acid and cocaine. This suggests that the biochemical approach in the therapy of the mental depressions, as in other psychiatric disorders, has just begun.

Chapter 15
LETTER TO A PSYCHIATRIST: CASE COMPLETED

You may be surprised to receive this letter. I am only one of many patients you have helped and have no special claim as a correspondent. You keep careful records on all of us and individualize us in terms of our problems and our needs. By means of these records and our weekly conversations, you build up a background of knowledge and gradually apply your skills to helping us help ourselves. Now I have reached the point where you can finish your record on me. I am a completed and, I believe, a successful case history. You have a right to feel some measure or professional satisfaction as you move on to take up the case of the next person on your waiting list.

Through the Looking Glass

But what about me? What do I think? What about my record of what has happened? This letter is my answer to these questions. I am more than a case history. I am a

143

sentient human being whose whole life has been changed for the better through your guidance. I want to speak from a patient's point of view and thus try to express to you my abiding sense of gratitude. Scientifically you must be aware of *what* you have given me and *how* you have given me what you have given me. But even though you do a wonderful job of putting yourself in your patient's place and seeing life through his or her eyes, you still are not one of us and cannot feel exactly as we feel. Because it is a good feeling, made possible by your skill and sympathy, I owe it to you to approximate it for you as closely as I can in words. Only then can you and I together write "case closed" on our mutual record.

To begin at the beginning, I must remember why I started coming to you nine months ago, 32 talks ago. As I look back, I am amazed that so much progress has taken place in less than three dozen visits. At the time, my problems loomed so large to me. I say that, even though I also felt that I already had considerable insight into them even before I turned to you. I had always been interested in mental health and psychiatry, had done a great deal of reading in the field, had helped others with their difficulties on occasion, and had gone as far as I could in analyzing my case. When I at last recognized that I was going around in circles and needed the aid of an objective counselor, I think I met the first requirement of successful psychotherapy; an acceptance of my need for help.

As I saw myself then, I was a more or less normal person with neurotic tendencies rather well under control and not noticeable to outsiders. In my middle years I was holding down a responsible public service position where I had received much public acclaim. I realized that people in general considered me an attractive and capable woman, young for my age, with a well-rounded family and professional life, rich in friends and achievements. I surmised that I would be the last person to be suspected of the maladjustments, anxieties, and conflicts which bothered me. Therein lay one of my difficulties. Partly because of people's expectations I had learned to keep up a front to the world and to bottle up my troubles inside myself. Small wonder that it was such a relief to talk to you openly and to try to get at the real self underneath the surface self.

Of course, you already knew a lot about my situation before I became your patient. This was due to an unusual set of circumstances. My teen-age son and daughter were already receiving psychiatric help from you. We all had in common a background of disturbed and unhappy family life. I had felt that as young people they should have the first chance to come to you and get straightened out and strengthened for adult life. They seemed to respond to the opportunity so well that I decided not to postpone taking the plunge myself. Among my many causes for gratitude to you I will always rank high the fact that you were willing to tackle three members of a family at once. It must have been quite an order and probably would have stumped the run-of-the-mill Practitioner. I understood that it was not the ordinary practice and I appreciated the opportunity and the responsibility of being an exception. I suppose that the inter-relatedness of our family problems had some clinical advantages for you to offset the disadvantages of being objective about each one of us in turn. Anyway, I had confidence in you from the very start and felt no reticence about telling you things I had never been able to tell anybody else.

Nobody had even known how unhappily married I was. The children, of course, suspected it, largely because they had been caught in the cross currents. But they were naturally more taken up with how it affected them. As they grew up, they had often resented, feared, and even hated their father for his set ways, his attempted dominance of their lives and his arbitrary and frequently cruel discipline through outbursts of temper and violence. As a mother, I inevitable revealed my alignment of sympathy with them, thus indicating to them an unsatisfactory wife-husband relationship. Actually I found it very hard to forgive him his lacks as a father and my bitterness poisoned our relationship the more I outwardly conformed to his patterns of behavior for the family.

What the children didn't suspect was that they were not the only "bone of contention" between my husband and myself; that our maladjustment had deep roots in the past. As I confessed to you in our first interview, I had married my husband wondering whether I really loved him. Because of a strict and over-protected family and school life, I had had little experience with men and was uncertain as to what love was and how one could recognize it. I was even more uncertain about myself and undoubtedly saw in my husband some sort of hoped-for security. Older by a good many years, widely travelled and well informed, he impressed me as a person of strength and ability on whom I could rely and whom I could undoubtedly come to love, even if not in the romantic story book way which my reason discarded anyway. For me it was a head-ruling-the-heart marriage, with the heads sadly mistaken in judgment.

What I found was a man dominated by fears of ill health and economic insecurity. He always seemed to be chronically ill or indisposed or fatigued and he was usually worrying about the future and jobs and my old age. I remember one day coming across the word "hypochondriac" in my reading and suddenly realizing that it applied to my husband. This was long before psychosomatic theories and parlance had developed. All these tendencies affected his disposition and mental outlook and had a direct bearing on our whole relationship. As you recognized, our serious sexual maladjustments were symptomatic of our total pat-

Added to basic lack of compatibility was the compulsion my husband has to re-shape my personality. He considered me too sensitive, too introverted, too much of a dreamer, too devoted to my friends. I needed to become more practical, more aware of the every day world and the struggle for survival, more efficient, more careful about saving money. Although I was too unsure of myself not to be sure he was incorrect, I nevertheless often rebelled and defended my values as expressed through my own personality pattern. This led to periodic quarrels, occasionally violent ones when I might run off and stay away for half a day or where he might get so angry that he would shake me or throw handy objects at me.

I was never fearful of my life in these crises, but I did come to feel more and more as if I were in prison. Even though my up-bringing had conditioned me against divorce and even though my lack of knowledge about worldly affairs made me timid about even investigating the possibility, I was leaning in this direction, after four years of unhappiness, when our first child was conceived. This took me by surprise and it was not a happy period for me, to understate the case. I felt more than ever as if I were caught in a net. I remember that I made one desperate struggle to disentangle myself when the children were four and six. I even left home for a few weeks. But my husband knew how to bring me to heel. He had told me that he would fight me in every court in the land to get custody of the children on the grounds that I wasn't a "fit mother" – a threat which again I was not armed to meet with practical knowledge and to which I was susceptible because of my constant worry about my inadequacies as a mother. To top it off, he wrote me that my little girl was ill and I flew home as fast as I could get there. From the time of her birth she had been delicate and I had been concerned about her. All my maternal instincts were aroused and I was back in the cage. But with a difference. This time I resolved that for the children's sake there were to be no more conflicts with my husband, and that I would do by best to fit myself to his pattern for the family peace.

But I reckoned without the violence in his nature. Increasingly as the children asserted their individuality, he tried to subdue and discipline them. When the boy especially showed signs of "stubbornness" his father's sudden wrath found expression in scoldings, deprivations, and beatings. More and more I became a mediator and pacifier, trying to smooth things over or even hide the knowledge of anything unpleasant from my husband so that he wouldn't blame the children. My own past need for individuality was forgotten and I hastened to be a model wife in order to propitiate him towards the children. During all these dreary years the obvious fact you showed me never once occurred to me: that he was using the children as tools to get his way and my attention, that actually I had three, not two children. At the time, all I recognized was that underneath I disliked him increasingly and felt guilty accordingly, especially since I sensed that in his way he loved me more than any other person in his life and was greatly dependent on me.

When the children were in their teens and showing the inevitable personality disorders for such home life, my cycle of resentment and guilt intensified. Sometimes I would get very depressed and blame myself for everything on the grounds that if I could have really loved him, none of these things might have happened. Yet I could see that violence springing from his inferiority feelings was a part of this nature and made it hard to love him.

In this confused ad anxious state of mind I turned to you. Because it had looked as if my husband might have a break down after one of his scenes of violence against our son, I had some years previous sought and found a full-time job requiring great expenditure of skill and energy. Although in some ways this work had offered me outlets for my own personality, I confessed to you that I had reached the end of my resources, with my candle not only burning at both ends but in danger of going out in the tempests of my life.

"But What Do You Feel?"

I not only poured out to you the story of my conflicts recapitulated above, but I added many details and examples which only you will even know and which I can never bring myself to put down on paper. But, of course, it took time – and great patience on your part – to dig up for our consideration all the hurt and pain and bitterness I had experienced. Even when I thought I was being most open and frank, you would show me that I was holding back. Too often I gave you my ideas, reasons, theories about things so that you constantly had to remind me, "But what do you *feel* about it?"

I began to see that I was still hiding my real feelings behind a lot of barriers. I would talk freely about family problems and my worries about the children, but I wouldn't talk freely about myself and my worries about myself. In other words, I was wrapped up in the children's needs so much that I couldn't recognize at first that I had needs of my own. It was very hard for me to recognize that I could actually help the children most by learning to help myself first. For years I had disciplined myself away from self-centeredness until my pattern of self-sacrifice had become unhealthy not only for myself but for its recipients.

What fascinated me at the time, and even now as I recall it, was the skillful way in which you gave me this insight. As a patient it is perhaps not up to me to evaluate your techniques, and it may even be that most of your patients are unaware of them. Yet, I wouldn't be writing this unusual kind of letter to you if I didn't happen to by analytical and introspective by nature, so please bear with me as I give you my worm's eye view on such matters.

If I had to summarize your technique in general, I would say it contained the genius of simplicity. You never expounded or explained at length, you merely dropped what appeared to be a casual remark or well-timed observations. But it was very much like planting seeds, with the sprouting taking place during the following days.

"What About You?"

in the case of my over concern about the children, for example, you met it by asking me the same question at different intervals – "But what about you?" I remember the first time you asked it I was quite startled. I didn't know what to answer because I wasn't in the habit of thinking about myself. The next time you asked me I had at least become aware of the fact that I, too, was a person who deserved some consideration. Once I had accepted that fact, I could see what you then pointed out: that I had been using the children as a smoke-screen to keep from a recognition of my own misery and loneliness. My idea had been that if you could help the children and I could help you help them by coming to you, then my own major problems would be solved. I couldn't have been more mistaken. Fortunately, I learned to render unto you the things that were yours, drop my anxieties about the children in your lap, and concentrate on myself.

"You Are Afraid, Aren't You?"

What kind of a person did I find when I turned the spotlight inward? There again I was in for some surprises. For example, I had always taken a certain amount of pride in considering myself a rather courageous person. It had seemed to me that I had stood up so well to the unhappy circumstances of my marriage and family for years that no one on the outside even suspected that I was suffering and unhappy. Yet one of your simple little questions knocked the prop out of this particular illusion. I remember that I was describing the likely violence which certain behavior on my part or the children's part might elicit from my husband. You looked at me searchingly and, quick as a flash, said, "You are afraid, aren't you?" Instinctively I had to agree. Rationally I then had to retrace my steps and find why it was that I had agreed. Together we worked out another new insight for me: that I had courage of a certain kind, yes, but that it was the courage of endurance rather that of initiative. As I reviewed with you what had been happening to me through the years, I began to see that I was very good when on the defensive, but very poor when on the offensive.

Naturally this discovery led me into further exploration. What was behind this pattern of endurance? Was I submitting to more than was reasonable to expect? If so, was it a pattern of self-punishment on my part, perhaps a perpetuation of early childhood patterns of guilt and resentment?

It is strange how quickly I came to see my whole personality pattern in this new light and how easily this perception led me into a new freedom of behavior. It is as if chains fell from my feet. I began of my own free will to do what I wanted to do in little ways regardless of my husband's disapproval, and gradually to do what I wanted to do in bigger ways. I found that courage breeds courage, and not only courage, but self-confidence and self-respect. Day by day I could almost feel the growing pains of a more positive attitude toward life and people, on the job and in the home. And what's more, it was fun to feel myself opening outwards instead of turned inwards. You showed me that I had to learn to like myself more that I had before I could genuinely like and enjoy others.

This is only another way of saying that my own worst enemy had been myself. Granted that I had had some unlucky circumstances and a bad break in my marriage, nevertheless the trouble did not lie in my husband or in anyone else who might give me a rough time. The trouble lay in myself if I allowed myself to be imposed upon. It was really up to me as to whether I wanted to be a strong person, operating from a sure center within myself.

This thought made a terrific impact on me. I had always believed in such noble sentiments as: "stone walls do not a prison make, nor iron bars a cage," and had always aimed to be "captain of my fate" and "master of my soul" in a spiritual sense at least. But now I knew that a lot of potential power had been dammed up inside me. For the first time you made me face the simple truth that no one could "push me around" if I didn't let them or even secretly want them or need them to do so. And what was really nice about all this was to see that the less I stayed a mouse, the more I liked people and they liked me--and this included my husband. As he came to respect my new independence, he treated me with more consideration which, in turn, made him feel less guilty and more able to come to terms not only with me but with himself. Thus we are gaining a certain modus vivendi in every-day life.

You will remember that at one stage in therapy I strongly considered the possibility of a divorce, or at least a separation, from my husband. I even left home for a few weeks to try it out and think it through. In a way I think you knew I had to take some such step in order to prove to myself that I was not in prison, that I was a free agent, and that nothing drastic would happen if I acted accordingly. I had imagined all sorts of dire happenings ranging from my husband's committing suicide to his directing violence against myself or the children in connection with my leaving. In fact, I was so fearful of the pistol he kept in his room that I did not dare tell him where I was living. Yet somehow I had to face up to these fears and master them through actual experience.

As usual, the actual experience lacked the terror of the imagined one. While my husband found the adjustment to my move hard to make, he learned a lot and thought a lot about the difficulties in our relationship and was the first to admit to me that it was the "best thing," that I had ever done. It shocked him into seeing things suddenly from my point of view.

"You Made the Choice This Time"

Although you never said so, I suppose you anticipated that I would work things out of my system to the point where I would return home again. But, as you pointed out in one of your classic sentences, "You made the choice yourself this time." And certainly in the succeeding months I have never once lost my sense of free choice. I came back with certain understandings with my husband in advance: that I would have some measure of independent life of my own to follow and develop my particular interests, that I would be able to manage my own income and expenditures without interference or criticism.

I suppose in one way we can never hope to have what might be called a good marriage. There are too many scars, too many incompatibilities. But we are learning to "live and let live." And we are preserving certain values in terms of family and community life which are probably more important to us at our age than if we were younger. All this is a lot and I have learned through you not to expect more than a lot.

"You Expect Too Much"

As you put it to me one day rather abruptly, "You expect too much of people." During the weeks that I digested your statement, I found that it applied to a whole range of people, including myself. I had not been aware beforethat I had a "perfectionist" on my hands and I really had to take her apart and put her together again in a more comfortable position. As a result, I have found it much easier to take a less tense and more relaxed attitude toward my job, my family, my friends, and my past, present, and future in general.

"You Are In the Present Now"

You certainly helped to relax me about the past. a perfectionist worries about past mistakes and a multitude of *if's*. Why did I not do this, would it not have been better if I had done that? Well, as you remarked, "Given the set of circumstances and you as you were you could hardly have done differently." To me this was more than a simple "don't cry over spilt milk" philosophy. It provided me with an acceptance of myself in the past as a stepping stone to the present. And there you were right ahead of me with your "thought for the week" when you reminded me, "That's all behind you, you are in the present now." Surely it must be a wonderful feeling for you as a psychiatrist when you help your patients to the point where they can drop off all the old burdens of grief and regret and really concentrate on the living, breathing present.

It was a happy thought for me that no one was doomed in a psychological sense any more than in a moral sense. I could see that my candle still had a lot of light left in it, and that it was up to me to hold it aloft and discover the world about me. As you suggested, an unsatisfactory marriage is not the end of a road unless one lets it be. As for emotional outlets, there are "all kinds of human relations possible with all kinds of people." Actually, I was in a particularly fortunate position since my daily work put me in contact with so many interesting and worthwhile individuals. For the outgoing rather than the ingrowing person, the world becomes a "Friends Unlimited" sort of proposition. Loneliness is a self-imposed martyrdom.

"Live With or Without"

Yet, at this very point I found one of my hardest hurdles. As I allowed my long-lost capacity for friendship to have its head again, I discovered a tendency to rely too much on those who symbolized it for me. I was intrigued by the fact that you refused to let me begin using my friends as props for my own security. You "with or without" slogan became quite a challenge to me. For my own good I had to learn to live "with or without" any particular person or persons. Granted that friendship was a universal need which must be constantly filled, too intense particularization of it could lead to dependence, hurt, disappointment, or what not, with the fluctuations or space, time, and circumstance. You helped me to see it very simple: that I could enjoy people more if I depended on any one person less, that I had to depend first and foremost on myself and my own inner strength.

This brought me full cycle back to this question of being a strong person. I had to work on it to bring my attitudes and feelings up to the level of my insight into its importance. But even I could tell from week to week that I was making progress. And, of course, you encouraged me in this belief. I tend to think that you use some magic system of "rewards" for your patients. I can recall that it was quite a red-letter day for me when you remarked to me after my 30th visit that I was a "much stronger person than before." I am convinced that such remarks are part of your effective technique, but I am also convinced that you sincerely mean what you say in such instances.

Patients are bound to trust you when you never speak lightly and without due consideration. They, in turn, know they must earn your commendations.

"Quite a Person"

Yet your personal evaluation wouldn't mean half as much unless they sprang from your objectivity. Perhaps that is the key to successful psychotherapy: a dynamic patient-therapist relationship marked by friendly understanding but within a framework of complete objectivity. Every human being should have the privilige of seeing himself through the eyes of a wise and fair person who will not take sides for or against him on an emotional basis. When you saw my weak points, I saw them too, because I knew you were not biased against me, and so they must be true. When you saw my strong points, again I saw them too, because I knew you were not biased in my favor. Thus when you looked reflectively at me one day and said, "You are quite a person, aren't you?" I had to agree. To an outside this would sound like gross conceit, yet an insider realizes that an honest appreciation of self is attained through "blood, sweat, and tears" and is held in the spirit of sincere humility and gratitude.

Creatures of Earth and Sky

Yes, there is no doubt in my mind that your counselling has helped me become a whole person for the first time in my life. It is as if I had gone from limping to walking to climbing, as if blinders had fallen from my eyes and I could behold the glorious light of day. All my life I have given lip-service to the creative possibilities in human nature, but because you have unlocked the unused resources within me, I now believe in people as never before. The strength in me is the strength of humanity.

That we are all bound one unto another, that we are all children of God, becomes an experience rather than an ideal.

How I wish that everybody could have the chance for the kind of experience and insight given to me. A person's right to mental health should be taken as much for granted as his right to physical health. Some day this will come, but meanwhile, I consider myself one of the lucky ones. In the public mind there are still many misconceptions about psychiatry as materialistic and psychiatrists as debunkers of traditional values. To me the kind of experience I have had is spiritual rather than materialistic, creative rather than disillusioning, stabilizing rather that destructive. I feel as if I were at long last rooted in the world of man and the world of God. You and I never discussed religion as such and, of course, never touched on your own personal life and outlook. Yet, I am convinced in my own mind that your work springs out of an essentially religious view of life. Please bear in mind that we have three witnesses in our family to the effect that you are motivated by faith, hope, and love for your fellow man. One of us might be mistaken, but three of us must be right! What can you do against a "cloud of witnesses?"

So now I can close this joint chapter with you, firm in the knowledge that the book of life still opens ahead. May you continue to do justice, love mercy, and walk humbly with your God, for the betterment of bewildered people. We are creatures of earth and must learn to find contentment upon it. But we are also born of flame and song, and are meant to grow and discover, aspire and attain. Let us dedicate our chapter to the mystery of man and the wonder of human personality.

www.ingramcontent.com/pod-product-compliance
Lightning Source LLC
Chambersburg PA
CBHW032020170526
45157CB00002B/791